Skincare

Secrets & Tips

Kimberly Hodge

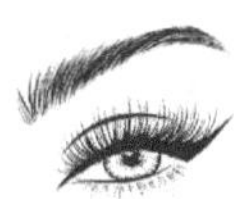

ISBN: 9798862887624
Cover design by: Kimberly Hodge
Printed in the United States of America

Disclaimer

The information provided in this book is for general informational purposes only and should not be considered as medical or professional advice. The author and publisher of this book are not dermatologists, cosmetologists, or medical professionals, and the tips and suggestions provided in this book are based on personal experiences and research.

Every individual's skin reacts differently to beauty, skincare, and cosmetic products and techniques. It is important to consult with a dermatologist or healthcare professional before implementing any new skincare or beauty routine, especially if you have pre-existing skin conditions, allergies, or sensitivities.

The author and publisher are not responsible for any adverse reactions, injuries, or damages that may result from the use or misuse of the information provided in this book. It is the reader's responsibility to carefully read product labels, perform patch tests, and seek professional guidance when necessary.

The recommendations and opinions expressed in this book are subject to change over time and may not always reflect the most current research or industry standards. The reader is advised to do their own research and exercise their own judgment when making decisions about their skincare and beauty regimen.

Furthermore, the author and publisher do not endorse or promote any specific beauty, skincare, or cosmetic products mentioned in this book. The inclusion of specific products, brands, or recommendations is for illustrative purposes only and does not constitute a personal endorsement. The reader is encouraged to conduct their own research and choose products that align with their personal needs and preferences.

In conclusion, while the information provided in this book is intended to be helpful and informative, it should not be considered as a substitute for professional advice. The reader assumes full responsibility for their skincare and beauty decisions and should always consult with a qualified professional for personalized recommendations.

Contents

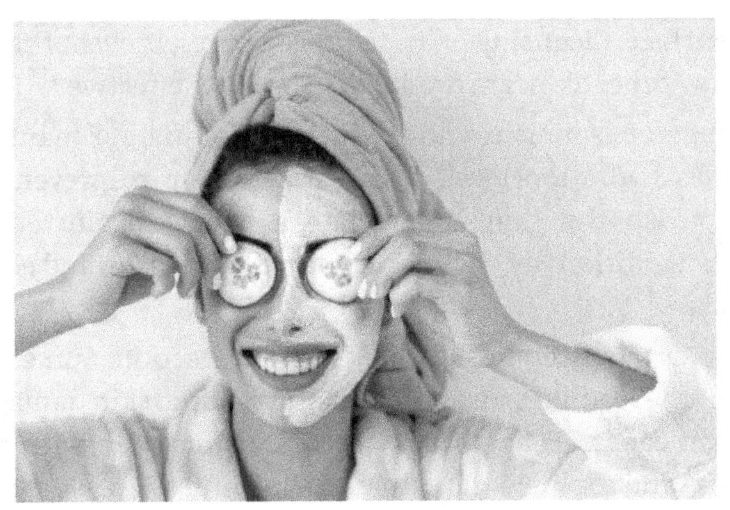

Introduction

Skincare is an essential aspect of our daily routines that focuses on maintaining the health and appearance of our skin. It involves the use of various products, techniques, and practices to protect, cleanse, moisturize, and nourish our skin. Skincare goes beyond just cosmetic purposes; it plays a vital role in maintaining the overall health and well-being of our largest organ, the skin.

The primary goal of skincare is to achieve and maintain healthy, clear, and radiant skin. It is important to understand that everyone's skin is unique and requires a personalized approach. Factors like skin type, concerns, and environmental conditions need to be considered when developing a skincare routine.

There are several key steps in a basic skincare routine that are recommended by experts. The first step is cleansing, which involves removing impurities, dirt, oil, and makeup from the skin's surface. Cleansing helps to unclog pores, prevent breakouts, and allow other skincare products to be more effective.

The next step is moisturizing, which is essential for maintaining the skin's hydration levels. Moisturizers help to prevent water loss, nourish the skin, and create a barrier against external irritants. Additionally, they can improve the texture and elasticity of the skin.

Another crucial step in skincare is sun protection. Sun exposure is one of the leading causes of premature aging, skin damage, and even skin cancer. Using broad-spectrum sunscreen with at least SPF 30 is vital to shield the skin from harmful UV rays.

Furthermore, exfoliation is an important step to incorporate into a skincare routine. It helps to remove dead skin cells, unclog pores, and enhance the skin's natural rejuvenation process. Exfoliating regularly can improve the skin's texture, minimize dullness, and promote a brighter complexion.

In addition to these basic steps, individuals may choose to incorporate targeted treatments based on their specific concerns. These could include serums, face masks, eye creams, and spot treatments to address issues such as acne, hyperpigmentation, fine lines, or dehydration.

Skincare is not just about applying products; it also involves adopting healthy lifestyle habits. Eating a balanced diet, staying hydrated, getting enough sleep, exercising regularly, and managing stress all contribute to healthy skin.

Skincare is a vital practice that helps to maintain and improve the health and appearance of our skin. By adopting a personalized skincare routine that includes cleansing, moisturizing, sun protection, exfoliation, and targeted treatments, we can promote healthy, glowing skin.

Alongside skincare products, incorporating healthy lifestyle habits ensures long-term benefits for our skin. Remember that consistency and patience are key, as it takes time to see the desired results.

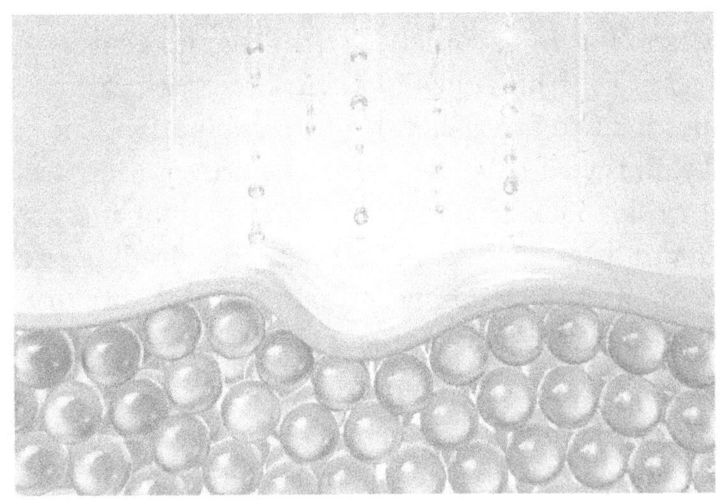

Chapter 1: Understanding Your Skin

Your skin is the largest organ of the body, and it plays a crucial role in protecting your internal organs from the outside world. It serves as a barrier against harmful bacteria, viruses, and other foreign substances, while also regulating your body temperature and preventing excessive moisture loss.

To truly understand your skin, it's important to know the three layers that make up: the epidermis, dermis, and subcutaneous tissue. The epidermis is the outermost layer and consists of several sublayers. It acts as a protective shield, shielding underlying layers from UV rays and other external factors. The dermis lies beneath the epidermis and contains collagen, elastin, blood vessels, and nerve endings. This layer gives your skin structure, elasticity, and strength. Finally, the subcutaneous tissue is made up of fat cells that provide insulation and act as a cushion for your organs.

Each person's skin is unique, with characteristics that vary due to genetics, ethnicity, and environmental factors. Common skin types include normal, dry, oily, combination, and sensitive. Normal skin is well-balanced, with a healthy appearance and few issues. Dry skin lacks moisture and can feel tight and itchy, while oily skin produces an excess of sebum, often leading to acne and a shiny complexion. Combination skin features both dry and oily areas, while sensitive skin is easily irritated and prone to redness and allergies.

Taking care of your skin involves understanding its specific type and needs. A consistent skincare routine is essential to maintain a healthy complexion. This typically includes cleansing, moisturizing, and protection from the sun. Cleansing helps remove dirt, oil, and impurities, while moisturizing ensures that the skin remains hydrated and nourished. Sun protection is crucial to shield your skin from harmful UV rays that can cause sunburn, premature aging, and even skin cancer.

Furthermore, it is important to be aware of how your skin reacts to different products and ingredients. Some individuals may have allergies or sensitivities to certain substances, causing adverse reactions like rashes or breakouts. Reading skincare product labels and understanding the ingredients they contain can help you make informed choices and minimize the risk of negative reactions.

Understanding your skin is the first step towards achieving and maintaining a healthy and radiant complexion. By knowing your skin type, developing a consistent skincare routine, and being mindful of the ingredients in the products you use, you can give your skin the care it deserves. Remember that everyone's skin is unique, so it's essential to listen to your skin's needs and adjust your skincare approach accordingly.

Skincare is an essential aspect of overall health and well-being. Our skin is the largest organ in the body and serves as a protective barrier against external elements such as pollutants, UV radiation, and harmful microorganisms. Therefore, taking care of our skin is crucial in maintaining its health and preventing various skin issues.

One of the key benefits of skincare is maintaining the skin's hydration. Moisturizing regularly helps to keep the skin soft, supple, and prevent dryness, which can lead to itchiness, irritation, and even flaking. Moreover, well-hydrated skin appears more youthful and radiant.

Skincare also plays a significant role in preventing premature signs of aging. As we age, our skin naturally loses collagen and elasticity, leading to the formation of wrinkles, fine lines, and sagging skin. However, practicing a consistent skincare routine that includes anti-aging products can help slow down the aging process and minimize the appearance of these signs. Ingredients like retinol, hyaluronic acid, and antioxidants are known to promote collagen production, strengthen the skin's structure, and combat the effects of environmental damage.

Furthermore, maintaining a proper skincare routine can help prevent and treat common skin conditions such as acne, hyperpigmentation, and inflammation. Regular cleansing and exfoliation can remove excess oil and dead skin cells, preventing clogged pores and breakouts. The use of targeted treatments and serums can also aid in reducing inflammation and promoting the healing of damaged skin.

Aside from the physical benefits, skincare also has a positive impact on our mental well-being. Taking the time to care for our skin can be a form of self-care and relaxation. Pampering ourselves with skincare rituals can help reduce stress, boost confidence, and foster a sense of self-love and acceptance.

Skincare is not just about superficial beauty but also about maintaining the health and vitality of our skin. Keeping our skin well-hydrated, protected from environmental stressors, and properly nourished can contribute to a vibrant and youthful appearance. Moreover, skincare promotes self-care and enhances our overall well-being. Therefore, incorporating a consistent skincare routine should be considered an essential part of our daily health regimen.

Skincare is essential for several reasons:

1. **Health:** Our skin is the body's largest organ and acts as a protective barrier against external elements like pollution, UV rays, and bacteria. Proper skincare helps maintain the skin's health, preventing issues such as infections, irritations, and allergies.

2. **Hydration:** Skincare products like moisturizers, serums, and lotions help replenish and maintain the skin's hydration levels. Adequately hydrated skin appears more plump, smooth, and radiant, while dehydrated skin can become dry, flaky, and prone to wrinkles.

3. **Anti-aging:** A consistent skincare routine can help slow down the aging process. Aging causes a decline in collagen and elastin production, leading to fine lines, wrinkles, and sagging skin. Skincare products containing ingredients like retinol, hyaluronic acid, and antioxidants can boost collagen production, improve elasticity, and reduce signs of aging.

4. **Sun protection:** Protecting our skin from harmful UV rays is crucial for preventing premature aging, pigmentation, sunburn, and reducing the risk of skin cancer. Applying sunscreen with a high SPF is a must, along with wearing protective clothing and seeking shade during peak sun hours.

5. **Confidence:** Taking care of your skin can greatly improve your self-esteem and confidence. When your skin looks and feels healthy, you are more likely to feel good about yourself and project that positive energy out into the world.

Overall, skincare is important for maintaining skin health, preventing issues, slowing down the aging process, protecting against sun damage, and promoting self-confidence. It is a self-care ritual that should be personalized according to individual skin type and concerns.

Benefits of maintaining a proper skincare routine

Maintaining a proper skincare routine is more than just a frivolous endeavor. It is a proactive approach towards taking care of your largest organ, the skin, and reaping the many benefits it offers. From improving the overall health and appearance of the skin to promoting self-confidence and slowing down the aging process, a proper skincare routine is an investment in one's wellbeing.

One of the main benefits of adhering to a skincare routine is the improvement in the skin's health. Regular cleansing, moisturizing, and exfoliating helps to remove dirt, oil, and dead skin cells from the surface, preventing clogged pores and breakouts. This can lead to a reduction in acne, blackheads, and skin irritation, making the skin clearer and healthier.

Another significant benefit of maintaining a skincare routine is the prevention of premature aging. Exposure to environmental pollutants and UV rays can lead to wrinkles, fine lines, and hyperpigmentation. However, with the help of skincare products such as sunscreen, antioxidants, and collagen-boosting serums, one can protect the skin against these external factors and slow down the aging process.

Furthermore, a proper skincare routine can greatly enhance one's self-confidence. When your skin looks and feels good, it can have a positive impact on your overall self-esteem. Clear, glowing skin can give you a healthy and youthful appearance, allowing you to feel more comfortable and confident in your own skin.

Lastly, a skincare routine is not just about the immediate benefits but also about long-term skin health. By taking preventive measures from early on, you can ensure that your skin stays vibrant and healthy in the future. Regular use of moisturizers, serums, and other skincare products can provide long-term hydration and nourishment, preventing dryness, dullness, and signs of aging.

Maintaining a proper skincare routine offers numerous benefits for both the health and appearance of the skin. From improving the overall health of the skin to preventing premature aging and boosting self-confidence, it is a worthwhile investment in yourself. So, take the time to establish a skincare routine that suits your specific needs and enjoy the positive impact it can have on your life.

Here are some key advantages:

1. **Healthy and glowing skin:** Following a regular skincare routine helps to keep your skin healthy,

nourished, and radiant. It helps to maintain the skin's natural balance and improve its overall appearance.

2. **Prevention of skin problems:** Regular skincare helps to prevent various skin problems like acne, breakouts, blemishes, and dullness. By removing dirt, oil, and dead skin cells, it reduces the chances of clogged pores and bacterial infections.

3. **Anti-aging effects:** A consistent skincare routine can help minimize the signs of aging, such as fine lines, wrinkles, and age spots. This is achieved through the use of targeted anti-aging products that promote collagen production and skin elasticity.

4. **Protection from environmental damage:** Skincare products like moisturizers, sunscreens, and antioxidants offer protection against harmful UV rays, pollution, and free radicals. This helps to minimize damage caused by external factors and maintain a healthier skin barrier.

5. **Improved self-confidence:** Clear, healthy skin can boost your self-confidence and self-esteem. When your skin looks and feels good, it can positively impact your overall mood and how you perceive yourself.

6. **Stress relief and relaxation:** Incorporating a skincare routine into your daily habits can be a calming and enjoyable self-care activity. Taking the time to cleanse, exfoliate, and moisturize can help relieve stress and promote relaxation.

Remember, everyone's skin is different, so it's important to choose products and routines that suit your specific needs. It's also recommended to consult with a dermatologist or skincare professional for personalized advice.

There are five main skin types, each with its own characteristics and needs. It's important to understand your skin type in order to properly care for it.

Here are the different skin types and their characteristics:

Normal Skin:

- Well-balanced and neither too oily nor too dry
- Smooth and even texture
- Small pores
- Few blemishes or imperfections

Dry Skin:

- Lack of moisture and can feel tight or itchy
- Dull and rough texture
- Fine lines and wrinkles may be more visible
- Small pores
- May experience flaking or peeling

Oily Skin:

- Excess production of sebum, causing a greasy or shiny appearance
- Thick and coarse texture
- Large, visible pores
- Prone to acne, blackheads, and breakouts

Combination Skin:

- Combination of oily and dry skin in different areas of

the face

- T-zone (forehead, nose, and chin) is oily, while cheeks may be dry or normal
- Pores may be larger in the oily areas

- Reacts easily to various triggers such as products, weather, or stress
- Prone to redness, irritation, and inflammation
- Can feel dry or itchy
- May develop rashes, hives, or breakouts when exposed to irritants

It's important to note that individuals may also have skin conditions or concerns on top of their skin type, such as acne, rosacea, or hyperpigmentation, which may require additional care. It's recommended to consult with a dermatologist to determine your specific skin type and address any concerns you may have.

Common skin concerns and issues

Common skin concerns and issues can vary depending on individual skin types and conditions. However, here are some of the most commonly experienced skin concerns:

1. **Acne:** This is a common skin condition characterized by the appearance of pimples, blackheads, and whiteheads. It is often caused by excess oil, bacteria, hormonal changes, or clogged pores.
2. **Dryness:** Dry skin lacks moisture and can be

characterized by flakiness, itchiness, and tightness. It can be caused by environmental factors, harsh skincare products, or underlying health conditions.

3. **Aging:** As we age, our skin naturally undergoes changes, including the appearance of wrinkles, fine lines, and loss of elasticity. These signs of aging can be influenced by factors such as sun exposure, genetics, and lifestyle choices.

4. **Hyperpigmentation:** This refers to the appearance of dark spots or patches on the skin, commonly caused by sun damage, hormonal changes, acne scars, or skin trauma.

5. **Sensitivity:** Some individuals have sensitive skin that reacts easily to certain ingredients or environmental factors, leading to redness, irritation, itching, or a stinging sensation.

6. **Oiliness:** People with oily skin tend to have excess sebum production, which can result in a shiny appearance, enlarged pores, and a higher risk of acne breakouts.

7. **Uneven skin tone:** Uneven skin tone is characterized by patches of skin that appear darker or lighter than the surrounding areas. It can be caused by sun exposure, hormonal changes, genetics, or certain skin conditions.

8. **Rosacea:** Rosacea is a chronic skin condition that causes redness, flushing, visible blood vessels, and sometimes acne-like bumps. It primarily affects the face and can be triggered by various factors, including sun exposure, hot temperatures, stress, and certain foods.

9. **Eczema:** Eczema, also known as atopic dermatitis, is

a chronic skin condition characterized by itchy, red, and inflamed skin. It is often triggered by allergies or irritants and can be managed with proper skincare routines and medication.

10. **Dark circles:** Dark circles around the eyes can be caused by various factors, including genetics, lack of sleep, stress, or allergies. They can make one appear tired or older and are often a cosmetic concern.

It is important to remember that seeking advice from a dermatologist or skincare professional is recommended for proper diagnosis and treatment of specific skin concerns or issues.

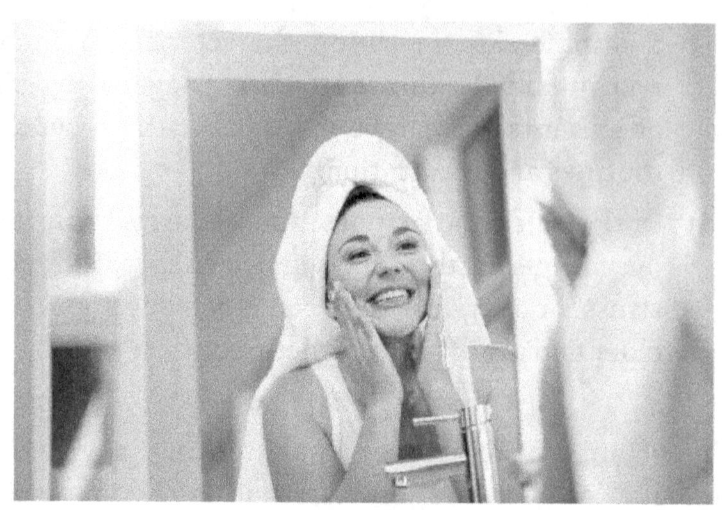

Chapter 2: Establishing a Skincare Routine

Establishing a skincare routine is essential in maintaining healthy, glowing skin. A consistent and effective skincare routine can help to improve the overall texture, tone, and appearance of the skin while also preventing various skin concerns such as acne, dryness, and signs of aging. With so many skincare products and options available in the market, it is crucial to understand and follow a routine that suits your specific skin type and concerns.

The first step in establishing a skincare routine is to identify your skin type. This can be done by observing your skin's behavior throughout the day and understanding its needs. Common skin types include oily, dry, combination, and sensitive. Knowing your skin type will help you choose the right products and ingredients that will address your skin concerns effectively.

Once you have determined your skin type, the next step is to cleanse your skin twice a day. Cleansing is essential to remove dirt, oil, and impurities that accumulate on the skin throughout the day. Choose a gentle cleanser that is suitable for your skin type and avoid harsh cleansers that can strip the skin of its natural oils. Massage the cleanser onto damp skin using gentle circular motions, and rinse thoroughly with lukewarm water.

After cleansing, it is important to moisturize your skin to keep it hydrated and nourished. Select a moisturizer that is appropriate for your skin type. If you have oily skin, opt for a lightweight, oil-free moisturizer. For dry skin, choose a richer, more hydrating formula. Apply the moisturizer onto cleansed skin, gently massaging it in upward motions until it is fully absorbed. Moisturizing not only helps to maintain the skin's moisture balance but also acts as a barrier to prevent water loss.

In addition to cleansing and moisturizing, incorporating a sunscreen with at least SPF 30 is crucial in protecting your skin from harmful UV rays. UV rays can cause premature aging, dark spots, and even skin cancer. Apply sunscreen generously on your face and exposed areas of your body every morning and reapply throughout the day if necessary. It is also recommended to use a broad-spectrum sunscreen that protects against both UVA and UVB rays.

Furthermore, a well-rounded skincare routine should include treatments and serums that target specific skin concerns. Whether it is acne, hyperpigmentation, or fine lines, there is a wide range of products available to address these concerns. Research and consult with a dermatologist or skincare professional to find the most suitable treatment options for your specific needs.

Lastly, establishing a skincare routine goes beyond just the products you use. Ensuring a healthy lifestyle can significantly contribute to the overall health and appearance of your skin. This includes practicing good hygiene, eating a balanced diet, staying hydrated, getting enough sleep, managing stress levels, and avoiding smoking and excessive alcohol consumption.

Establishing a skincare routine is vital for achieving and maintaining healthy, radiant skin. By identifying your skin type, selecting appropriate products, and following a consistent and personalized routine, you can nourish your skin, address specific concerns, and protect it from external damage. Remember, diligence and patience are key to seeing long-term results and enjoying the benefits of a well-cared-for complexion.

A. Cleansing

Importance of proper cleansing techniques

Proper cleansing is essential for maintaining healthy skin. Here are a few reasons why proper cleansing techniques are important:

a. Removes dirt and impurities: Throughout the day, our skin accumulates dirt, bacteria, pollutants, and dead skin cells. Cleansing helps to remove these impurities, preventing clogged pores and breakouts.

b. Balances oil production: Cleansing helps to remove excess oil from the skin, preventing an overly oily complexion. It also helps to regulate oil production, which is important for those with oily or combination skin.

c. Enhances absorption of skincare products: Cleansing ensures that the skin is clean and free from barriers like dirt and oil. This allows other skincare products, such as serums and moisturizers, to penetrate effectively and provide maximum benefits.

d. Promotes cell renewal: Regular cleansing helps to stimulate cell turnover, leading to a healthier, more radiant complexion. It also helps to unclog pores, preventing the formation of blackheads and whiteheads.

Choosing the right cleanser for your skin type

There are various types of cleansers available in the market, designed for different skin types. Here are some tips for choosing the right cleanser for your skin type:

a. Oily or acne-prone skin: Look for gel or foaming cleansers that help to control oil and unclog pores. Ingredients like salicylic acid or tea tree oil can be beneficial for reducing acne.

b. Dry or sensitive skin: Opt for creamy or lotion-based cleansers that are gentle and hydrating. Avoid harsh ingredients like sulfates and fragrances, as they can further dry out or irritate the skin.

c. Combination skin: Look for a mild, pH-balanced cleanser that can effectively cleanse without stripping the skin's natural oils. Gel or foam cleansers can be suitable for combination skin.

d. Normal skin: Consider yourself lucky! You have more flexibility in choosing a cleanser. Look for a gentle cleanser that suits your preferences.

e. Consider your lifestyle: If you wear heavy makeup, a double cleansing method using an oil-based cleanser followed by a water-based cleanser may be more effective for thoroughly removing makeup residue.

Remember, everyone's skin is unique, so it may take some trial and error to find the perfect cleanser for your skin type. If you're unsure, consult with a dermatologist or skincare professional for personalized advice.

B. Exfoliating

Benefits of exfoliation

Removes dead skin cells: Exfoliating helps to slough off dead skin cells from the surface of the skin, allowing for new, healthy skin cells to regenerate. This can result in smoother, brighter, and more radiant skin.

Improves skin texture: Regular exfoliation can help to improve the texture of the skin by minimizing the appearance of roughness, dry patches, and uneven skin tone.

Enhances product absorption: By removing the layer of dead skin cells, exfoliation allows for better absorption of skincare products such as moisturizers, serums, and treatments, which can maximize their effectiveness.

Evens out skin tone: Exfoliating can help to fade dark spots, hyperpigmentation, and acne scars, resulting in a more even complexion.

Prevents clogged pores: Regular exfoliation can help to unclog pores, reducing the risk of acne breakouts and blackheads by getting rid of trapped oil and debris.

Different types of exfoliants and when to use them

Physical exfoliants: These include scrubs, brushes, or loofahs that physically scrub away dead skin cells. They are effective in removing surface-level debris. Use physical exfoliants 1-3 times a week, depending on your skin's sensitivity.

Chemical exfoliants: These include ingredients such as alpha-hydroxy acids (AHAs) like glycolic acid or lactic acid, and beta-hydroxy acids (BHAs) like salicylic acid. They work by dissolving the bonds between dead skin cells, making them easier to remove. Chemical exfoliants are generally gentler and can be used more frequently, depending on the product's instructions.

Enzyme exfoliants: These contain natural enzymes (typically derived from fruits) that break down the proteins that hold dead skin cells together. They are usually mild and suitable for sensitive skin types. Follow the product instructions for usage frequency.

It's important to note that exfoliation should be tailored to your skin type and sensitivity. If you have sensitive or acne-prone skin, it's advisable to consult with a dermatologist or skincare professional to determine the most suitable exfoliation routine for you.

Purpose of toners

The main purpose of toners is to balance the pH level of the skin after cleansing. They are designed to remove any remaining traces of dirt, oil, and makeup that may have been missed during the cleansing process. Toners can also help to shrink the appearance of pores, hydrate the skin, and provide added nutrients and antioxidants.

Selecting the right toner for your skin

Choosing the right toner for your skin type is essential to ensure that it effectively addresses your specific needs.

Here are a few tips to help you select the right toner:

a. Identify your skin type: Determine whether your skin is oily, dry, combination, or sensitive. This will help you narrow down your options and choose a toner that is suitable for your specific skin needs.

b. Consider the ingredients: Look for toners that contain ingredients that are beneficial for your skin type. For example, if you have oily skin, opt for a toner that contains ingredients like witch hazel or salicylic acid, which can help control excess oil. If you have dry skin, choose a toner that is hydrating and contains ingredients like hyaluronic acid or glycerin.

c. Avoid toners with harsh ingredients: Stay away from toners that contain alcohol or other harsh ingredients, as they can dry out and irritate the skin. Opt for gentle, alcohol-free toners that are suitable for daily use.

d. Patch test before use: If you have sensitive skin or are trying a new toner, it's always a good idea to do a patch test before applying it to your entire face. Apply a small amount of the toner on your inner arm or behind your ear and wait for 24 hours to check for any adverse reactions.

e. Consult a skincare professional: If you're unsure about which toner is best for your skin, consider consulting a dermatologist or skincare professional who can provide personalized recommendations based on your specific concerns and needs.

Remember, everyone's skin is unique, so it may take some trial and error to find the perfect toner for your skin. Be patient, and don't be afraid to adjust your skincare routine as needed.

D. Moisturizing

Importance of moisturizers in skincare

Moisturizers are an essential part of any skincare routine as they help to nourish and hydrate the skin. Here are some reasons why moisturizers are important:

a. Hydration: Moisturizers help to trap water in the skin, preventing it from becoming dry and parched. They replenish moisture lost throughout the day due to environmental factors, such as sun exposure, wind, and pollution.

b. Skin barrier protection: Moisturizers create a protective barrier on the skin's surface, preventing water loss and shielding the skin from external irritants. This barrier function helps to maintain the skin's overall health and integrity.

c. Anti-aging properties: Regularly using moisturizers can help to reduce the appearance of fine lines and wrinkles. Adequately moisturized skin appears plump and firm, giving a more youthful complexion.

d. Soothing benefits: Moisturizers often contain ingredients that calm and soothe the skin, such as aloe vera or chamomile. These properties make moisturizers particularly beneficial for individuals with sensitive or irritated skin.

e. Enhances skin texture: Dry skin often feels rough and flaky. Moisturizers help to smoothen and soften the skin's texture by adding moisture and improving the overall appearance.

Choosing the appropriate moisturizer for your skin type

When it comes to choosing a moisturizer, it is crucial to consider your specific skin type.

Here are some general guidelines:

a. Dry skin: Look for moisturizers with hydrating and emollient properties. Ingredients like hyaluronic acid, shea butter, and ceramides can help to replenish moisture and improve dry skin. Opt for richer, cream-based moisturizers.

b. Oily skin: Lightweight, oil-free moisturizers or gel-based formulas are ideal for oily skin types. Look for products with non-comedogenic labels to prevent clogging of pores. Ingredients like salicylic acid or mattifying agents can also help control excess oil.

c. Combination skin: For combination skin, a moisturizer that balances hydration without clogging pores is essential. Consider using different moisturizers for different areas of the face. For example, a lightweight moisturizer for the oily T-zone and a slightly heavier one for the drier cheeks.

d. Normal skin: Lucky enough to have normal skin? You can choose a wide range of moisturizers based on your preference, from lightweight lotions to slightly heavier creams. Look for ingredients that nourish and hydrate the skin.

e. Sensitive skin: Opt for fragrance-free and hypoallergenic moisturizers specifically formulated for sensitive skin. Look for soothing ingredients like aloe vera, chamomile, or oat extract.

Keep in mind that everyone's skin is unique, so experimentation may be necessary to find the perfect moisturizer for your specific needs. It's also essential to consider other factors such as climate, season, or any specific skin concerns you may have.

Understanding the importance of sun protection

Sunscreen is a crucial component of sun protection as it helps to shield your skin from harmful ultraviolet (UV) rays emitted by the sun. UV rays can cause various damage to the skin, including sunburn, premature aging, and an increased risk of skin cancer. It's essential to understand the importance of using sunscreen to safeguard your skin from these harmful effects.

Selecting the right sunscreen and proper application

When selecting a sunscreen, here are a few considerations to keep in mind:

a. SPF (Sun Protection Factor): Choose a sunscreen with a broad spectrum, which protects against both UVA and UVB rays. Look for an SPF of 30 or higher, as this indicates better protection against the sun's harmful rays.

b. Formulation: Sunscreens come in different forms such as creams, lotions, sprays, gels, or sticks. Choose one that suits your preferences and skin type. Creams and lotions may be more moisturizing, while sprays or gels are lighter and easier to apply.

c. Skin type: Consider your skin type when selecting a sunscreen. If you have oily or acne-prone skin, choose a non-comedogenic or oil-free sunscreen that won't clog pores. For sensitive skin, opt for a fragrance-free and hypoallergenic formula.

d. Water-resistance: If you plan to swim or perspire, opt for a water-resistant sunscreen that maintains its effectiveness even after getting wet. However, keep in mind that these sunscreens should still be reapplied every two hours.

Proper application of sunscreen is as important as choosing the right one. Follow these tips:

a. Apply enough sunscreen: Use at least one ounce (about a shot glass) of sunscreen to cover your entire body. Don't forget commonly neglected areas like the ears, back of the neck, and tops of your feet.

b. Apply 15-30 minutes before sun exposure: Give the sunscreen ample time to absorb into your skin and form a protective barrier before stepping out into the sun.

c. Reapply regularly: Even if a sunscreen claims to be water-resistant, it's essential to reapply every two hours or immediately after swimming or sweating heavily.

d. Don't forget about lip protection: Apply a lip balm with SPF to protect your lips from sun damage.

In summary, understanding the importance of sun protection and selecting the right sunscreen, while ensuring proper application, are crucial steps in safeguarding your skin from the sun's harmful rays.

F. Extras

Face masks and their benefits

Face masks are a popular addition to skincare routines because of their numerous benefits for the skin. Here are some common types of face masks and their specific benefits:

a. Hydrating masks: These masks are formulated to deeply moisturize and hydrate the skin, making them ideal for those with dry or dehydrated skin. They often contain ingredients like hyaluronic acid, aloe vera, or glycerin.

b. Exfoliating masks: These masks help to remove dead skin cells and unclog pores, leaving the skin smoother and brighter. They usually contain ingredients such as AHAs (alpha hydroxy acids) or enzymes that gently slough off the top layer of the skin.

c. Clay masks: Clay masks are great for oily or acne-prone skin as they absorb excess oil and impurities from the pores. They can help to tighten the skin and reduce the appearance of pores. Some common types of clay used in masks are bentonite, kaolin, or French green clay.

d. Sheet masks: Sheet masks are pre-cut masks made from cloth or paper soaked in a serum. They are convenient to use and deliver a concentrated dose of ingredients to the skin. Sheet masks are available for different purposes like brightening, hydrating, firming, or soothing the skin.

Serums, oils, and other additional skincare products

Serums, oils, and other additional skincare products are often used to target specific skin concerns or provide extra nourishment to the skin. Here are some common types and their benefits:

a. Serums: Serums are lightweight and highly concentrated formulas that typically contain active ingredients like vitamins, antioxidants, or hyaluronic acid. They are designed to penetrate deeply into the skin and provide specific benefits such as hydration, brightening, or anti-aging effects. Serums are usually applied after cleansing and toning the skin, but before moisturizing.

b. Facial oils: Facial oils are moisturizing products that can benefit various skin types, including dry, dehydrated, or mature skin. They provide intense hydration, nourishment, and help to seal in moisture. Some popular facial oils include jojoba oil, argan oil, rosehip oil, or marula oil. Facial oils can be used alone or mixed with other products like moisturizers or serums.

c. Spot treatments: Spot treatments are designed to target specific blemishes like pimples, acne spots, or dark spots. These products often contain ingredients like salicylic acid, benzoyl peroxide, or niacinamide, which help to reduce inflammation and promote the healing process.

d. Eye creams: Eye creams are specifically formulated for the delicate skin around the eyes. They help to reduce the appearance of fine lines, puffiness, and dark circles. Eye creams often contain ingredients like retinol, peptides, or hyaluronic acid.

Remember, it's important to choose skincare products that are suitable for your skin type and address your specific concerns. You can consult with a dermatologist or skincare professional for personalized recommendations.

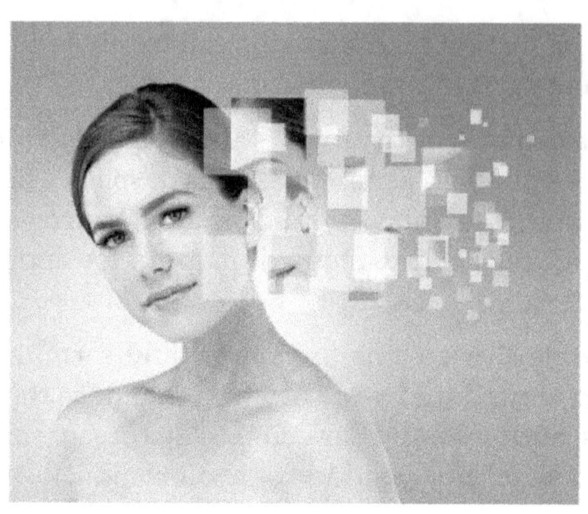

Chapter 3: Targeting Specific Skin Concerns

Targeting specific skin concerns requires understanding the underlying causes and developing a customized skincare routine. Whether it's acne, wrinkles, hyperpigmentation, or dryness, addressing the root of the problem is essential for effective results. With the right knowledge and targeted products, you can tackle any skin concern and achieve a healthier and more radiant complexion.

Acne is a common skin concern that affects people of all ages. It is usually caused by excess oil production, clogged pores, and bacterial growth on the skin. To target acne, it's important to use products that contain ingredients like salicylic acid or benzoyl peroxide. These ingredients penetrate the pores, unclog them, and eliminate acne-causing bacteria. Incorporating a gentle cleanser, exfoliator, and spot treatment into your routine can help control breakouts and prevent new ones from forming.

Another common concern is the appearance of wrinkles and fine lines. Aging, sun exposure, and loss of collagen contribute to the formation of these visible signs of aging. Targeting this concern involves using products with ingredients like retinol, which stimulates collagen production and promotes cell turnover. Additionally, incorporating a moisturizer enriched with hyaluronic acid can help plump the skin and reduce the appearance of wrinkles. Protecting the skin from sun damage with a broad-spectrum sunscreen is also crucial in preventing further wrinkles.

Hyperpigmentation, or dark spots on the skin, can be caused by sun damage, hormonal changes, or post-inflammatory hyperpigmentation (PIH) from acne or wounds. Treating this concern involves using products with ingredients like vitamin C, kojic acid, or niacinamide. These ingredients have brightening properties that help reduce the appearance of dark spots and even out the skin tone. Sun protection is vital in preventing the dark spots from getting darker and to avoid new ones from forming.

Dryness and dehydration can make the skin dull, flaky, and prone to premature aging. To address this concern, it's important to use products that provide intense hydration and restore the skin's moisture barrier. Look for moisturizers that contain ingredients like ceramides, hyaluronic acid, or glycerin. Additionally, incorporating a hydrating serum or facial oil in your skincare routine can help nourish and replenish the skin, leaving it soft, supple, and glowing.

Targeting specific skin concerns requires a tailored approach. Identifying the root causes, choosing the right ingredients, and establishing an effective skincare routine can help address acne, wrinkles, hyperpigmentation, and dryness. Consistency and patience are key since visible improvements may take time. By taking care of your skin and using the right products, you can effectively target these concerns and achieve a healthier, more radiant complexion.

Causes and treatment options

Treatment options for acne-prone skin include:

a) Topical treatments: Products containing ingredients like benzoyl peroxide, salicylic acid, or retinoids can help unclog pores, reduce inflammation, and prevent bacterial growth.

b) Oral medications: In severe cases, dermatologists may prescribe antibiotics or hormonal medications to control acne.

c) Professional treatments: Procedures like chemical peels, microdermabrasion, or laser therapy can be effective for managing acne-prone skin.

d) Lifestyle changes: Consistent skincare routine, avoiding picking or squeezing pimples, and adopting a balanced diet can also contribute to reducing acne.

Proper skincare routine for acne-prone skin

a) Cleansing: Use a gentle, non-comedogenic cleanser to cleanse your face twice a day (morning and night). Avoid harsh cleansers that can strip the skin of its natural oils, as this can trigger increased oil production. Look for cleansers with active ingredients like salicylic acid to unclog pores.

b) Exfoliation: Incorporate exfoliation into your routine but be cautious not to overdo it. 1-2 times a week is usually sufficient to remove dead skin cells and unclog pores. Opt for chemical exfoliants like salicylic acid or glycolic acid instead of harsh physical scrubs.

c) Moisturizing: Apply a lightweight, oil-free, non-comedogenic moisturizer that won't clog pores. Even acne-prone skin needs hydration to maintain a healthy skin barrier. Look for moisturizers with soothing ingredients like aloe vera or hyaluronic acid.

d) Spot treatment: If you have active breakouts, consider using a targeted spot treatment containing benzoyl peroxide or salicylic acid to help reduce inflammation and promote healing.

e) Sun protection: Protect your skin from harmful UV rays by applying a broad-spectrum sunscreen with an SPF of 30 or higher. Look for non-comedogenic formulas to avoid clogging your pores.

f) Makeup: Choose non-comedogenic, oil-free makeup products. Avoid heavy foundations and opt for lightweight, breathable formulas. Remember to remove your makeup thoroughly before bedtime.

g) Consistency and caution: Stick to your skincare routine consistently and be patient. It may take time to see significant improvements. Avoid picking or squeezing pimples, as this can worsen inflammation and potentially lead to scarring.

Remember, it's always a good idea to consult with a dermatologist to determine the best treatment plan for your specific skin type and severity of acne.

B. Aging skin

Understanding the aging process

- Skin aging is a natural process that occurs over

time due to both intrinsic (genetic) and extrinsic (environmental and lifestyle) factors.

- Intrinsic aging is inevitable and is characterized by a decrease in collagen and elastin production, leading to thinner and more fragile skin.

- Extrinsic aging is influenced by external factors like sun exposure, smoking, pollution, poor nutrition, and stress, which can accelerate the aging process.

Tips for anti-aging skincare

- Protect your skin from the sun: Daily use of sunscreen with at least SPF 30 is essential to prevent photoaging. Remember to apply it even on cloudy or winter days.

- Adopt a gentle skincare routine: Use mild cleansers that do not strip away natural oils. Avoid harsh scrubs that can cause irritation and dryness.

- Moisturize effectively: Use moisturizers rich in hyaluronic acid, glycerin, or ceramides to restore hydration and maintain a healthy skin barrier.

- Use products with retinoids: Retinoids, such as retinol or prescription-strength versions like tretinoin, can stimulate collagen production, reduce wrinkles, and improve skin texture. Start slowly to minimize potential irritation and always use sunscreen when using retinoids.

- Include antioxidants in your routine: Antioxidants like vitamin C, vitamin E, or green tea extracts can help protect against free radicals and oxidative stress, which accelerate aging.

- Hydrate from within: Drink plenty of water and maintain a well-balanced diet rich in fruits, vegetables, whole grains, and lean proteins to provide essential nutrients for healthy skin.
- Get enough sleep: Lack of sleep can contribute to premature aging. Aim for 7-8 hours of quality sleep per night to allow your skin to regenerate.
- Stay hydrated and avoid smoking: Hydration and avoiding smoking contribute to overall skin health and can help slow down the aging process.
- Consider professional treatments: If desired, options like chemical peels, microdermabrasion, laser therapy, or dermal fillers can be discussed with a dermatologist to address specific concerns.

It's important to note that while these tips can help in maintaining healthy skin and potentially slow down the aging process, they may not reverse significant signs of aging. Consulting with a dermatologist or skincare professional can provide personalized advice for your specific needs.

C. Dry skin

Common causes of dryness

Some common causes of dry skin include:

- **Weather conditions:** Cold and dry air can strip the skin of its natural moisture, leading to dryness.

- **Hot showers and baths:** Taking long showers or baths in hot water can remove the natural oils from the skin, causing dryness.

- **Harsh soaps and cleansers:** Using products that contain strong chemicals or fragrances can strip the skin of its natural oils and lead to dryness.

- **Age:** As people age, their skin produces less oil, making it more prone to dryness.

- **Certain medical conditions:** Conditions like eczema, psoriasis, and thyroid disorders can cause dry skin.

Skincare tips for dry skin

If you have dry skin, here are some tips to help keep it hydrated and relieve dryness:

- **Use a gentle cleanser:** Opt for mild, fragrance-free cleansers that won't strip away the natural oils in your skin. Avoid using hot water and instead use lukewarm water for washing your face and body.

- **Moisturize regularly:** Apply a thick, hydrating moisturizer after cleansing to lock in moisture and keep your skin hydrated. Look for moisturizers that contain natural oils, shea butter, or ceramides.

- **Protect your skin:** Protect your skin from harsh weather conditions by wearing appropriate clothing like hats and gloves, and use a moisturizing sunscreen with at least SPF 30 when going outside.

- **Use a humidifier:** To combat dryness caused by indoor heating or air conditioning, use a humidifier at home to add moisture to the air.

- **Avoid harsh products:** Steer clear of products that contain alcohol, fragrances, or other irritating ingredients that can further dry out your skin.
- **Exfoliate gently:** Use a gentle exfoliant once or twice a week to remove dead skin cells and allow better absorption of moisturizers. Avoid harsh scrubbing and opt for chemical exfoliants with ingredients like alpha-hydroxy acids (AHAs).
- **Stay hydrated:** Drink plenty of water throughout the day to keep your body and skin hydrated from within.
- **Avoid long, hot showers:** Limit your shower or bath time and use lukewarm water instead of hot water to prevent further drying out of your skin.

Remember, if your dry skin becomes severe, doesn't improve with home remedies, or is accompanied by other concerning symptoms, it's best to consult a dermatologist for further evaluation and treatment options.

D. Oily skin

Causes of excess oil production

- **Hormonal changes:** During adolescence, the body undergoes hormonal changes, leading to increased sebum (oil) production.
- **Genetics:** Some individuals naturally produce more oil than others, which can be inherited.

- **Environment:** Hot and humid climates can stimulate the sebaceous glands to produce more oil.

- **Over washing or harsh cleansing:** Stripping the skin of its natural oils can actually lead to increased oil production as the skin tries to compensate.

- **Certain skincare or makeup products:** Some products can clog the pores and cause the skin to produce more oil as a result.

Managing oily skin with the right skincare routine

- **Cleanse properly:** Use a gentle, oil-free cleanser to remove excess oil and impurities from the skin twice a day. Avoid harsh scrubs or cleansers with strong chemicals that can irritate the skin and trigger even more oil production.

- **Use toner:** Applying a toner after cleansing can help remove any residue left behind and minimize the appearance of pores.

- **Moisturize:** Even oily skin needs hydration. Look for oil-free, lightweight moisturizers that are specifically formulated for oily skin.

- **Exfoliate regularly:** Exfoliating helps remove dead skin cells, unclog pores, and maintain a balanced oil production. Use a gentle exfoliator or a chemical exfoliant containing salicylic acid.

- **Use oil-absorbing products:** Look for products like blotting paper or oil-absorbing sheets to help control shine throughout the day without stripping the skin of its natural oils.

- **Avoid heavy makeup:** Opt for lightweight, oil-free, and non-comedogenic makeup products that won't clog the pores. Avoid applying too much makeup, as it can trap oil and dirt on the skin.

- **Use clay masks:** Applying a clay mask once or twice a week can help absorb excess oil and impurities from the skin.

Remember, it's important to consult with a dermatologist if you have persistent oily skin concerns or if the problem worsens despite following a proper skincare routine.

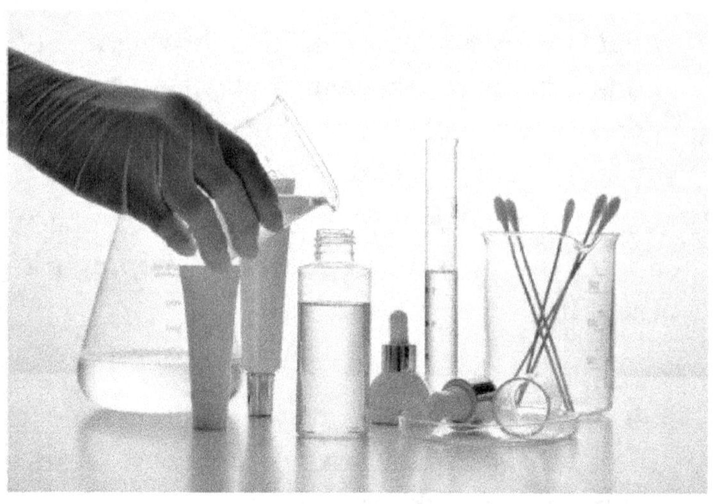

Chapter 4: Skincare Ingredients

Skincare ingredients play a crucial role in the health and appearance of our skin. The skin is the largest organ of our body, and it acts as a protective barrier against external aggressors. A well-formulated skincare product with effective ingredients can nourish, repair, and replenish the skin, resulting in a radiant complexion and a more youthful appearance.

One of the key benefits of skincare ingredients is their ability to hydrate and moisturize the skin. Ingredients like hyaluronic acid, glycerin, and ceramides are known for their excellent moisturizing properties. They help to attract and retain moisture, thus preventing dryness, flakiness, and dullness. Proper hydration not only keeps the skin soft and supple but also helps to maintain its elasticity and reduce the appearance of fine lines and wrinkles.

Skincare ingredients can also provide significant anti-aging benefits. Ingredients like retinol, peptides, and antioxidants such as vitamin C, vitamin E, and green tea extract help to stimulate collagen production, improve skin elasticity, and reduce the signs of aging. These powerful ingredients can diminish the appearance of wrinkles, fine lines, dark spots, and uneven skin tone, promoting a more youthful and rejuvenated complexion.

Another crucial aspect of skincare ingredients is their ability to repair and protect the skin from environmental damage. Ingredients like niacinamide, vitamin C, and antioxidants have been proven to combat free radicals, which are unstable molecules that can damage the skin cells and accelerate the aging process. Regular use of products containing these ingredients can help to prevent oxidative stress, protect against sun damage, and promote a healthy skin barrier.

Skincare ingredients also target specific skincare concerns such as acne, hyperpigmentation, and sensitivity. For acne-prone skin, ingredients like salicylic acid, benzoyl peroxide, and tea tree oil work effectively to unclog pores, reduce inflammation, and control breakouts. Hyperpigmentation can be treated with ingredients like hydroquinone, kojic acid, and vitamin C, which inhibit melanin production and promote a more even and radiant skin tone. Skincare ingredients suitable for sensitive skin, such as aloe vera, chamomile, and oat extract, can soothe and calm irritated skin, reducing redness and inflammation.

Skincare ingredients are not just marketing gimmicks but vital components of an effective skincare routine. They provide hydration, anti-aging benefits, repair, protection, and address specific skin concerns. It is essential to choose products with well-researched and clinically proven ingredients to ensure their efficacy and safety. Regular use of skincare products with the right ingredients can help us achieve and maintain healthy, radiant, and youthful-looking skin.

A. Essential skincare ingredients

Hyaluronic acid, retinol, vitamin C, etc.

Hyaluronic acid, retinol, and vitamin C are three popular skincare ingredients known for their various benefits in promoting healthy and youthful skin. Each compound has unique properties that make them effective in addressing specific skin concerns.

Hyaluronic acid is a substance naturally found in the human body, primarily in the skin, eyes, and connective tissues. It is known for its powerful hydration properties. As a skincare ingredient, hyaluronic acid works by attracting and retaining moisture, resulting in plump and moisturized skin. It helps to restore the skin's moisture barrier, improving the appearance of fine lines and wrinkles and providing a smoother, more supple complexion.

Retinol, or vitamin A, is a potent anti-aging ingredient that has been widely studied and recognized for its ability to smooth wrinkles, even out skin tone, and improve overall texture. Retinol stimulates collagen production, which helps to increase skin elasticity and reduce the visibility of fine lines and wrinkles. Additionally, it can promote the shedding of dead skin cells, unclogging pores and reducing the occurrence of acne.

Vitamin C, also known as ascorbic acid, is a powerhouse antioxidant that protects the skin from environmental damage caused by free radicals. It helps to brighten the skin by inhibiting the production of melanin, reducing the appearance of dark spots, and promoting a more even skin tone. Vitamin C also boosts collagen production, improving skin firmness and reducing the signs of aging. It can also enhance the skin's natural defense mechanisms, improving its ability to repair itself and maintain a healthy and radiant complexion.

It is important to note that while these three ingredients offer a multitude of benefits, they may not be suitable for everyone, and caution should be exercised when incorporating them into skincare routines. Individuals with sensitive or reactive skin should start with low concentrations and gradually increase usage to minimize the risk of irritation. Consulting with a dermatologist or skincare professional can also provide valuable insights and guidance on how to best incorporate these ingredients into a skincare routine for maximum effectiveness.

Parabens, sulfates, artificial fragrances, etc.

Parabens, sulfates, and artificial fragrances are three commonly found ingredients in personal care and cosmetic products. Knowing about these ingredients can help you make informed decisions when it comes to choosing the right products for yourself.

Parabens are a group of preservatives used in many skincare and beauty products. They are effective at preventing the growth of bacteria, fungi, and other microorganisms. However, there has been some concern about their potential health effects. Parabens have been found to mimic the hormone estrogen, and there is evidence linking them to hormonal disruption and various health issues. While research is ongoing, many individuals choose to avoid products that contain parabens as a precautionary measure.

Sulfates, on the other hand, are a class of detergents commonly used in shampoos, body washes, and cleansers to create a foaming effect. They are effective at removing dirt, oil, and impurities from the skin and hair. However, sulfates can also strip away natural oils, leaving the skin and scalp dry and irritated. Some people with sensitive skin or certain hair conditions like dryness or color-treated hair may choose to avoid products containing sulfates to prevent further irritation or damage.

Artificial fragrances are ingredients added to personal care products to provide a pleasant scent. They can be found in products ranging from perfumes and colognes to lotions, soaps, and shampoos. While these fragrances may smell enticing, they are often made up of a combination of synthetic chemicals. Some individuals may find that these artificial fragrances cause skin irritation, allergies, or headaches. To mitigate this, many people prefer to opt for products that are fragrance-free or scented with natural, plant-based ingredients.

To cater to the growing demand for cleaner and more natural products, many companies now offer paraben-free, sulfate-free, and fragrance-free options. These products are formulated without these potentially problematic ingredients, making them appealing to those who prefer to avoid them. Additionally, there has been a rise in the availability of natural and organic personal care products that utilize alternative preservation methods and use botanical or essential oil-based fragrances.

Ultimately, the choice to use products with parabens, sulfates, and artificial fragrances is a personal one. It's important to be aware of any potential health concerns and to consider your individual needs and preferences. Reading product labels, conducting research, and consulting with healthcare professionals can all aid in making informed choices about the personal care products you use on your body.

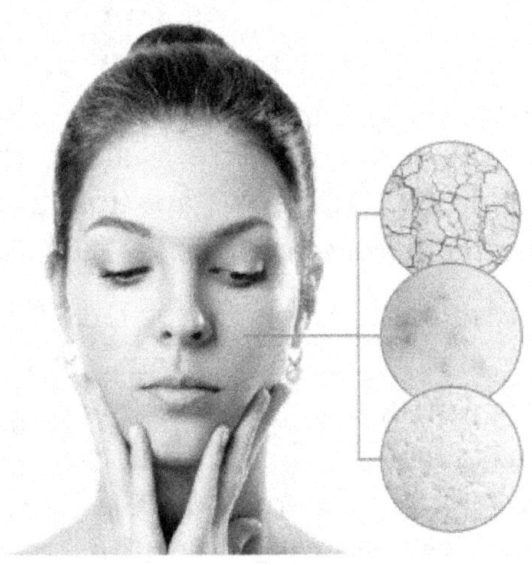

Chapter 5: Lifestyle Factors Impact

Lifestyle factors play a crucial role in maintaining healthy skin. Our daily habits, choices, and behaviors significantly impact the condition and appearance of our skin. Here, we will explore some key lifestyle factors and their impact on skin health.

One of the most significant lifestyle factors that affect the skin is diet. What we consume directly affects the overall health of our skin. A diet rich in fruits, vegetables, whole grains, and lean proteins provides essential nutrients, vitamins, and antioxidants that promote skin health. Antioxidants help protect the skin from damage caused by free radicals, which can speed up the aging process and lead to skin problems like wrinkles and fine lines. Conversely, a diet high in processed foods, sugars, and unhealthy fats can lead to inflammation and result in skin issues such as acne and dullness.

Another lifestyle factor that influences skin health is exercise. Regular physical activity promotes good blood circulation, which brings oxygen and nutrients to the skin cells, nourishing them from within. Exercise also helps flush out toxins through sweat, which can lead to clearer and healthier skin. Additionally, exercise reduces stress levels, and since stress is known to contribute to various skin problems like acne flare-ups and eczema, regular exercise can improve skin conditions.

Sleep is another crucial lifestyle factor that impacts skin health. During sleep, our body goes into repair and regeneration mode, and this applies to our skin as well. Lack of adequate sleep can lead to increased stress levels, which in turn can result in skin issues like acne and breakouts. Moreover, insufficient sleep can disrupt the skin's natural healing process, leading to a dull complexion, dark circles, and premature aging. Therefore, getting enough quality sleep is essential for maintaining healthy skin.

Protecting the skin from the sun's harmful UV rays is another critical lifestyle factor. Sun exposure not only causes sunburn but can also result in long-term damage to the skin, such as wrinkles, age spots, and an increased risk of skin cancer. Using sunscreen with a high SPF, wearing protective clothing, and seeking shade during peak sun hours are all essential for preserving the health and appearance of the skin.

Lastly, managing stress is vital for overall skin health. Chronic stress can lead to hormone imbalances, which can trigger acne breakouts and other skin problems. Additionally, stress can impair the skin's barrier function, leading to increased sensitivity, redness, and inflammation. Engaging in stress-reducing activities such as meditation, yoga, or hobbies can have a positive impact on the skin.

Lifestyle factors have a significant impact on the health and appearance of our skin. By adopting a healthy diet, regular exercise routine, getting enough sleep, protecting our skin from the sun, and managing stress levels, we can promote optimal skin health and enjoy a vibrant and glowing complexion.

A. Diet and hydration

Maintaining a healthy diet and staying properly hydrated can greatly impact the health of your skin. A diet rich in fruits, vegetables, whole grains, and healthy fats can provide essential vitamins, minerals, and antioxidants that promote skin health. It is also important to drink plenty of water throughout the day to keep your skin hydrated and flush out toxins.

B. Stress management and its influence on skin health

Stress can have a negative impact on your skin's appearance and overall health. When you are stressed, your body releases stress hormones like cortisol, which can lead to increased oil production, breakouts, and other skin issues. Managing your stress levels through techniques like meditation, exercise, and finding time for relaxation can help improve your skin's condition.

C. Exercise and its effects on the skin

Regular exercise not only provides numerous health benefits for your body but also has positive effects on your skin. Exercise improves blood circulation, which ensures that oxygen and nutrients are delivered to your skin cells, resulting in a healthy, glowing complexion. Additionally, sweating during exercise helps to unclog pores and flush out toxins, which can improve overall skin clarity. However, it's important to shower and cleanse your skin after exercising to remove any sweat and bacteria buildup.

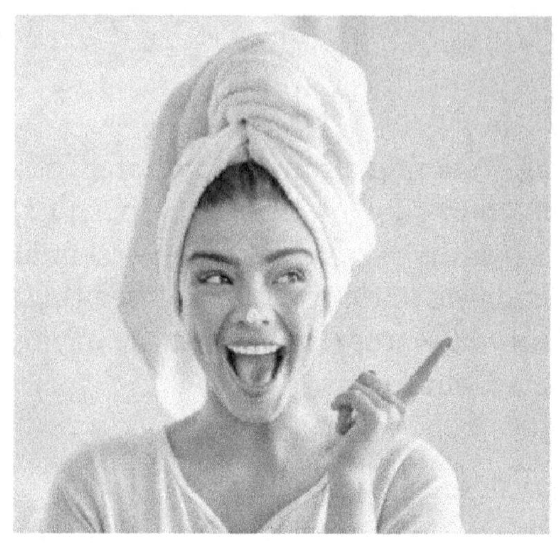

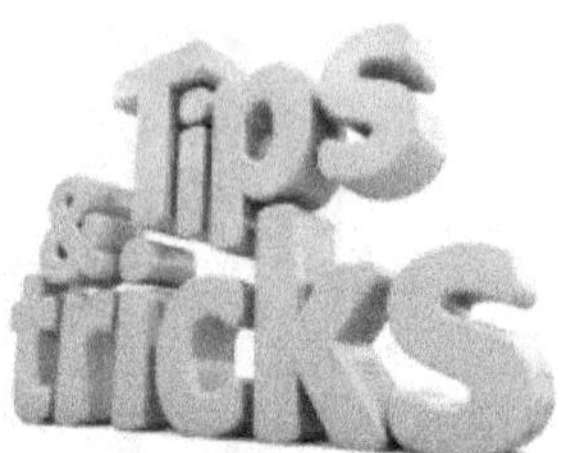

Chapter 6: Skincare Tips

Skincare is essential at all ages as it helps to maintain the health and appearance of our skin. However, the needs of our skin change as we grow older.

Let's explore some skincare tips for different age groups:

A. Skincare routine for teenagers

A skincare routine for teenagers should focus on keeping the skin clean, hydrated, and protected.

Here's a basic skincare routine that can be followed daily:

1. **Cleansing:** Use a gentle facial cleanser twice a day, once in the morning and once before bed. Look for a mild,

non-comedogenic cleanser that is suitable for your skin type.

2. **Toning:** After cleansing, use a toner to remove any remaining impurities and restore the pH balance of your skin. Look for alcohol-free toners to avoid drying out your skin.

3. **Moisturizing:** Apply a lightweight, oil-free moisturizer to hydrate your skin. This step is important even if you have oily or acne-prone skin, as it helps maintain a healthy moisture balance.

4. **Sun protection:** Apply a broad-spectrum sunscreen with SPF 30 or higher every day, even on cloudy days. This will help protect your skin from harmful UV rays and prevent premature aging.

5. **Spot treatment:** If you have acne or blemishes, apply a spot treatment containing ingredients like benzoyl peroxide or salicylic acid to help clear up breakouts. Use it only on affected areas, as spot treatments can be drying.

6. **Weekly exfoliation:** Once or twice a week, use a gentle exfoliator to remove dead skin cells and unclog pores. Be careful not to over-exfoliate, as it can irritate the skin.

7. **Face masks:** Incorporate a face mask into your routine once a week to address specific skincare concerns. Look for masks that target acne, oily skin, dryness, or other skin issues you may have.

Remember, everyone's skin is different, so it's important to adjust your skincare routine to suit your own needs. Additionally, if you have any specific skin concerns or conditions, it's a good idea to consult with a dermatologist for personalized guidance.

In your 20s: This is the time when most people enjoy youthful, radiant skin. To maintain this glow, it's important to establish a skincare routine that focuses on prevention and protection. Cleanse your skin twice a day with a gentle cleanser and exfoliate once or twice a week to remove dead skin cells. Moisturize daily and wear sunscreen with at least SPF 30 to protect against harmful UV rays. Don't forget to remove your makeup before going to bed to allow your skin to breathe and regenerate overnight.

In your 30s: As you enter your 30s, your skin starts to show signs of aging. Hydration becomes crucial to retain elasticity and prevent wrinkles. Incorporate an anti-aging serum into your routine, rich in ingredients like hyaluronic acid and vitamin C, to promote collagen production and diminish fine lines. Additionally, consider using eye creams to address under-eye bags and dark circles. Don't skip regular exfoliation as it helps to promote cell turnover, keeping your skin bright and smooth.

Here are some skincare tips to follow during this stage:

1. **Follow a consistent skincare routine:** Establish a daily skincare routine that includes cleansing, toning, and moisturizing. Use products suitable for your skin type.

2. **Use sunscreen daily:** Sun protection is crucial to prevent premature aging and protect against harmful UV rays. Opt for a broad-spectrum sunscreen with an SPF of 30 or higher.

3. **Exfoliate regularly:** Regular exfoliation helps remove dead skin cells and promotes cell turnover. This can be done using chemical exfoliants like AHAs or BHAs or

with gentle physical exfoliants.

4. **Hydrate your skin:** Keep your skin hydrated by drinking plenty of water throughout the day. This helps maintain skin elasticity and prevent dryness.

5. **Include antioxidants in your routine:** Antioxidants like vitamin C and E can help protect your skin from free radicals and environmental damage. Look for serums or moisturizers containing these ingredients.

6. **Take care of your eye area:** The skin around the eyes is delicate and prone to fine lines. Use an eye cream or gel to hydrate and minimize the appearance of dark circles and puffiness.

7. **Incorporate retinol:** Consider adding a retinol product to your skincare routine. Retinol helps improve fine lines, uneven skin tone, and texture over time. Start with a low concentration and gradually increase as your skin tolerates it.

8. **Manage stress:** Stress can take a toll on your skin, leading to breakouts and dullness. Practice stress management techniques like meditation, yoga, or regular exercise to keep your skin healthy.

9. **Avoid over-exfoliating or over-drying your skin:** Be mindful of not over-exfoliating or using harsh products that strip the skin's natural oils. This can lead to irritation, excessive dryness, and breakouts.

10. **Get enough sleep:** A good night's sleep is essential for skin rejuvenation and repair. Aim for 7-8 hours of quality sleep each night.

Remember, everyone's skin is unique, so it's important to listen to your skin's needs and adjust your skincare routine accordingly. Consulting with a dermatologist can also provide personalized advice for your specific skin concerns.

In your 40s and beyond: In your 40s and beyond, your skin may start to show signs of aging such as fine lines, wrinkles, and loss of elasticity.

As you age, your skin's needs change even more. Focus on deeply hydrating your skin with moisturizers that contain hyaluronic acid and ceramides to replenish moisture and strengthen the skin's barrier. Consider adding retinol or other prescription creams containing ingredients like peptides and antioxidants to help combat fine lines, wrinkles, and age spots. It's also important to remember that a healthy lifestyle, including a balanced diet, regular exercise, and ample sleep, plays a significant role in maintaining youthful-looking skin.

Here are some skincare tips to help you maintain a healthy and youthful complexion:

1. **Moisturize:** Use a rich and nourishing moisturizer both morning and night to hydrate your skin and help reduce the appearance of fine lines. Look for ingredients like hyaluronic acid, which helps retain moisture and plump up the skin.

2. **Sun protection:** Protect your skin from the sun's harmful rays by wearing sunscreen with at least SPF 30 every day, even on cloudy days. Sun damage can accelerate visible signs of aging, so it's crucial to shield your skin.

3. **Retinol/Retinoids:** Consider incorporating retinol or

retinoid products into your skincare routine. These vitamin A derivatives can help improve fine lines, wrinkles, and uneven skin texture. Start with a low concentration and gradually increase usage to avoid irritation.

4. **Antioxidant-rich products**: Use skincare products packed with antioxidants, such as vitamins C, E, and niacinamide. These ingredients help neutralize free radicals and protect against environmental damage.

5. **Exfoliation**: Regular exfoliation can help remove dead skin cells and promote cell turnover, revealing a brighter and smoother complexion. Choose gentle exfoliants like chemical exfoliators with AHAs or BHAs instead of harsh physical scrubs, which can be too abrasive.

6. **Eye care**: Pay special attention to the delicate skin around the eyes. Incorporate an eye cream that addresses specific concerns like puffiness, dark circles, and fine lines.

7. **Hydration from within**: Stay hydrated by drinking plenty of water throughout the day. Proper hydration is essential for skin health and can help maintain a youthful appearance.

8. **Healthy lifestyle**: Adopting a healthy lifestyle can also positively impact your skin. Get enough sleep, manage stress levels, exercise regularly, and follow a balanced diet rich in fruits, vegetables, and omega-3 fatty acids.

9. **Consistency and patience**: Remember that skincare results take time, so be consistent with your routine and patient with the process. Commit to a skincare regimen and stick to it to see long-term improvements.

Additionally, it's always a good idea to consult with a dermatologist or skincare professional to tailor a skincare routine that suits your specific needs and concerns.

Regardless of age, certain skincare practices remain important for everyone. Always protect your skin from the sun by wearing sunscreen, even on cloudy days. Stay hydrated by drinking plenty of water to keep your skin plump and hydrated from the inside out. Avoid smoking and limit alcohol consumption as they accelerate skin aging. Finally, remember to be gentle with your skin; avoid harsh products and excessive scrubbing that can cause irritation and damage.

Remember, everyone's skin is unique, so it's essential to listen to your skin's needs and adjust your skincare routine accordingly. Regularly consult with a dermatologist who can provide personalized advice based on your specific skin concerns and age.

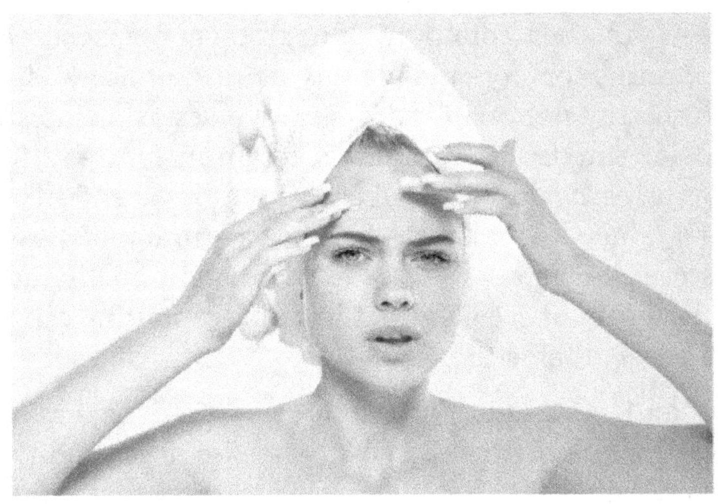

Chapter 7: Problem-Solving Skincare

Problem-solving skincare refers to the use of specific skincare products and routines to address various skin concerns and issues. These concerns can range from acne breakouts and dryness to redness and signs of aging. The goal of problem-solving skincare is to target these specific concerns and find effective solutions to improve the overall health and appearance of the skin.

One of the most common skin concerns is acne breakouts. Problem-solving skincare for acne typically involves using products that are specifically formulated to treat and prevent pimples. This may include cleansers with salicylic acid to unclog pores and control oil production, spot treatments containing benzoyl peroxide to kill bacteria, and moisturizers that do not clog pores or exacerbate breakouts. Additionally, regular exfoliation can help to remove dead skin cells and prevent the formation of acne-causing bacteria.

Dryness is another common skin problem, especially during colder months or for individuals with naturally dry skin. Problem-solving skincare for dryness involves using moisturizers that provide intense hydration and retain moisture in the skin. Ingredients like hyaluronic acid and ceramides are often included in these products to replenish the skin's natural moisture barrier and restore suppleness and elasticity. Additionally, adding a hydrating serum or facial oil to the skincare routine can provide an extra boost of moisture.

Redness and sensitivity are concerns often experienced by individuals with sensitive skin or those who have conditions like rosacea or eczema. Problem-solving skincare for redness typically involves using gentle, soothing products that help to calm and balance the skin. Ingredients like aloe vera, chamomile, and green tea are known for their anti-inflammatory properties and can help reduce redness and irritation. Avoiding harsh products and ingredients, such as alcohol-based toners or fragrances, is also essential for preventing further irritation.

Signs of aging, such as wrinkles, fine lines, and loss of firmness, are concerns for many individuals. Problem-solving skincare for aging skin often includes ingredients like retinol, peptides, and antioxidants, which help to stimulate collagen production, improve skin texture, and reduce the appearance of wrinkles. Additionally, using SPF every day is crucial to protect the skin from further damage caused by sun exposure, which can contribute to premature aging.

Problem-solving skincare involves tailoring a skincare routine and using specific products to address individual skin concerns. Whether it's treating acne, combating dryness, reducing redness, or fighting signs of aging, there are various skincare solutions available. It is essential to identify and understand your specific skin concerns to choose appropriate products and develop an effective problem-solving skincare routine that meets your needs.

Dealing with specific skin concerns such as acne scars and dark spots can be frustrating, but there are several methods you can try to help improve the appearance of your skin.

Here are some tips and suggestions:

1. **Cleanse your skin properly:** Start by using a gentle cleanser to remove dirt, excess oil, and impurities from your skin. Avoid harsh cleansers that may strip your skin's natural oils, as this can lead to further irritation and inflammation.

2. **Exfoliate regularly:** Exfoliation helps to remove dead skin cells and promote cell turnover, which can help fade acne scars and dark spots over time. Choose a gentle exfoliator with ingredients like salicylic acid or glycolic acid, which can help brighten and smooth your skin.

3. **Use products with active ingredients:** Look for skincare products that contain active ingredients known for their skin-lightening and scar-fading properties. Some common ingredients include hydroquinone, kojic acid, vitamin C, retinol, and niacinamide. However, always patch test new products and consult a dermatologist before using them to ensure they are suitable for your skin type.

4. **Protect your skin from the sun:** Sun exposure can make acne scars and dark spots more prominent. Therefore, it's essential to use sunscreen with a broad-spectrum SPF of 30 or higher, even on cloudy days.

Additionally, wearing hats and protective clothing can further shield your skin from harmful UV rays.

5. **Consider professional treatments:** If home remedies and over-the-counter products aren't providing the desired results, you may want to explore professional treatments. Consult with a dermatologist or skincare specialist who can recommend treatments such as chemical peels, microdermabrasion, laser therapy, or dermal fillers, depending on your specific concerns.

6. **Adopt a healthy lifestyle:** Good overall health can contribute to healthy skin. Maintain a well-balanced diet rich in fruits, vegetables, and antioxidants. Get regular exercise, stay hydrated, and manage stress levels. These factors can help improve your skin's overall appearance and aid in the healing process.

Remember, consistency is key when dealing with skin concerns. Results may not be immediate, and it may take some time to notice a significant improvement. Be patient, follow a skincare routine that works for you, and don't hesitate to seek professional advice if needed.

B. Troubleshooting skincare issues

Here are some common concerns and possible solutions:

1. **Acne:** If you're dealing with breakouts, consider using products with salicylic acid or benzoyl peroxide to help clear the pores and reduce inflammation. It's also essential to maintain a consistent cleansing routine and avoid touching your face excessively.

2. **Dry Skin:** For dry skin, focus on hydrating and moisturizing your skin. Look for products with

ingredients like hyaluronic acid, ceramides, and glycerin. Avoid using harsh cleansers or hot water when washing your face, as they can strip away moisture. Applying a moisturizer immediately after cleansing, while your skin is still slightly damp, can help lock in hydration.

3. **Oily Skin:** If you have oily skin, look for lightweight, oil-free products that won't clog your pores. Consider using a gentle cleanser twice a day and incorporating a toner with ingredients like witch hazel or tea tree oil to help control excess oil. You may also find it helpful to use a clay or charcoal mask once or twice a week to draw out impurities and absorb oil.

4. **Hyperpigmentation:** To tackle dark spots or hyperpigmentation, incorporate products with ingredients like vitamin C, niacinamide, or alpha arbutin into your skincare routine. These ingredients can help brighten the complexion and fade dark spots over time. Additionally, always remember to apply sunscreen during the day to prevent further pigmentation and protect your skin from sun damage.

5. **Sensitivity or Redness:** If you have sensitive skin or often experience redness, prioritize gentle, fragrance-free skincare products with soothing ingredients like aloe vera, chamomile, or green tea extract. Avoid harsh exfoliants or irritating ingredients and perform patch tests on new products before using them on your face.

Remember, everyone's skin is unique, so it's essential to listen to your skin and adjust your routine accordingly. If you're struggling with severe or persistent issues, it's always a good idea to consult a dermatologist for professional guidance.

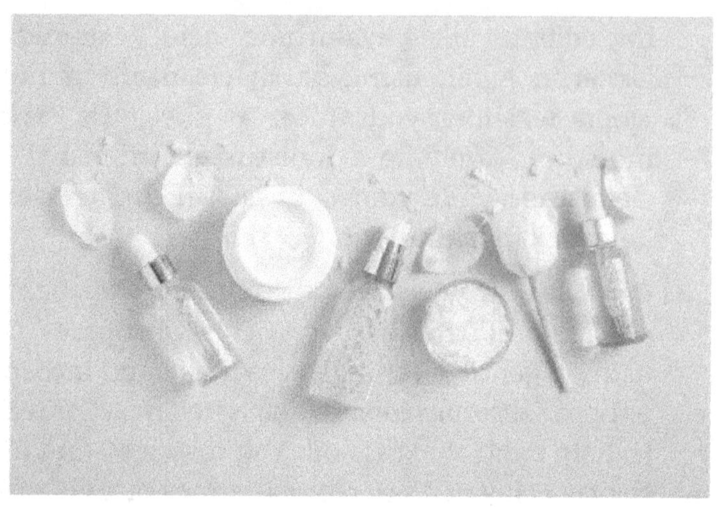

Chapter 8: Incorporating Natural Skincare

Incorporating natural and DIY skincare into your beauty routine can offer numerous benefits for your skin and overall health. Natural skincare involves using products made from naturally derived ingredients, such as plant extracts, essential oils, and organic compounds. DIY skincare, on the other hand, involves creating your own skincare products using natural ingredients found in your kitchen or pantry.

One of the primary advantages of natural skincare is that it minimizes the exposure to harmful chemicals and artificial ingredients commonly found in commercial beauty products. Many store-bought skincare products contain ingredients like parabens, sulfates, and synthetic fragrances, which can lead to skin irritations, allergies, and long-term health issues. By using products made from natural ingredients, you reduce the risk of these adverse effects and provide your skin with the nutrients it needs to stay healthy.

DIY skincare allows you to have full control over the ingredients you use, allowing you to personalize your products according to your skin's specific needs. For example, if you have dry skin, you can create a nourishing face mask using ingredients like avocado, honey, and yogurt. These ingredients are known for their moisturizing properties and can help replenish hydration and softness to your skin. Similarly, if you have oily or acne-prone skin, you can make a DIY toner using witch hazel, tea tree oil, and distilled water to help balance oil production and reduce breakouts.

Moreover, incorporating natural and DIY skincare is often a more budget-friendly option compared to purchasing high-end skincare products. Many natural ingredients can be found in your kitchen or local grocery store, making them much more affordable than expensive beauty brands. Creating your own skincare products also allows you to experiment and find the perfect combination of ingredients that work best for your skin without breaking the bank.

In addition to the benefits for your skin, natural and DIY skincare can also have positive environmental impacts. Commercial beauty products often come in plastic containers that contribute to pollution and waste. By making your own skincare products using natural ingredients, you can reduce your plastic consumption and overall environmental footprint. Furthermore, when you opt for natural products, you support sustainable farming practices and promote the use of renewable resources.

Incorporating natural and DIY skincare into your beauty routine can be a wonderful way to nourish and care for your skin without exposing it to harmful chemicals. By using natural ingredients, you provide your skin with the nutrients it needs, enjoy a personalized experience, save money, and contribute to a healthier environment.

So why not give it a try and start exploring the wonders of natural and DIY skincare today?

There are several benefits of using natural ingredients in skincare:

1. **Safety:** Natural ingredients are typically less likely to cause skin irritation or adverse reactions compared to synthetic ingredients, making them suitable for sensitive skin types.

2. **Nourishment:** Natural ingredients often contain high levels of essential nutrients, vitamins, and minerals that can provide nourishment to the skin. These nutrients can help replenish and rejuvenate the skin, promoting a healthier complexion.

3. **Hydration:** Many natural ingredients, such as aloe vera, honey, and hyaluronic acid, have excellent hydrating properties. They can help to moisturize the skin, improving its texture and preventing dryness.

4. **Antioxidant properties:** Various natural ingredients, such as green tea extract, vitamin C, and rosehip oil, possess antioxidants. These antioxidants can help protect the skin from environmental damage, including UV radiation and pollution, and minimize the appearance of aging signs like wrinkles and fine lines.

5. **Gentle and soothing:** Natural ingredients like chamomile, cucumber, and oatmeal are known for their soothing properties. They can help calm irritated skin, reduce redness, and provide relief from conditions such as acne, eczema, or rosacea.

6. **Sustainability and eco-friendly:** Many natural skincare brands promote sustainable practices by using responsibly sourced ingredients, practicing ethical farming, and minimizing environmental impact. By choosing products with natural ingredients, you are supporting an eco-friendlier approach to skincare.

It is important to note that natural ingredients can also cause allergies or sensitivities in some individuals. It's always recommended to do a patch test and consult with a dermatologist if you have any concerns or specific skin conditions.

B. Homemade skincare remedies and recipes

Here are some homemade skincare remedies and recipes that you can try:

1. **Honey and oatmeal face mask:** Mix 1 tablespoon of honey with 2 tablespoons of finely ground oatmeal. Apply the mixture to your face and leave it on for 15-20 minutes. Rinse off with warm water. This mask can help soothe and moisturize the skin.

2. **Coconut oil moisturizer:** Apply a small amount of coconut oil to your face and body after showering. Coconut oil is a natural moisturizer that can help hydrate and nourish the skin.

3. **Green tea toner:** Brew a cup of green tea and let it cool. After cleansing your face, apply green tea to your skin using a cotton pad. Green tea contains antioxidants that can help reduce inflammation and refresh the

skin.

4. **Cucumber eye gel:** Blend half a cucumber and strain the juice. Mix the cucumber juice with 1 tablespoon of aloe vera gel. Apply a small amount of this mixture to your under-eye area and leave it on for 10-15 minutes. Cucumber has a cooling effect and can help reduce puffiness and dark circles.

5. **Brown sugar and olive oil scrub:** Mix 1 tablespoon of brown sugar with 1 tablespoon of olive oil. Gently massage the mixture onto your face or body in circular motions. Rinse off with warm water. This scrub can help exfoliate and soften the skin.

Remember to patch test any new skincare products or ingredients on a small area of your skin before applying them to your face or body to check for any potential allergies or reactions.

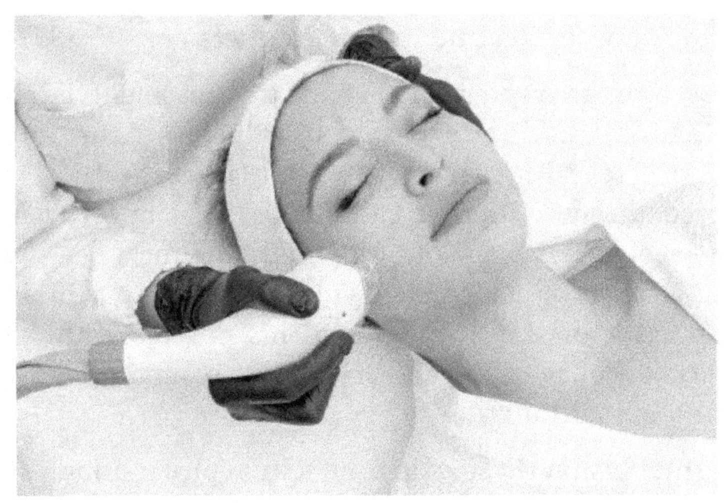

Chapter 9: Professional Skincare Treatments

Professional skincare treatments are a vital part of maintaining healthy and radiant skin. These treatments are performed by trained professionals who have extensive knowledge about different skin types and conditions. They use advanced techniques and high-quality products to address specific concerns and provide long-lasting results.

One popular professional skincare treatment is a facial. A facial involves a thorough cleansing of the skin to remove dirt, oil, and impurities. The esthetician then uses techniques such as exfoliation to remove dead skin cells and promote cell turnover. This process helps to unclog pores and improve the texture and tone of the skin. Additionally, a facial often includes a soothing massage to relax facial muscles and improve blood circulation. This not only helps to promote a healthy glow but also aids in the absorption of other treatments and products.

Another common professional skincare treatment is chemical peels. Chemical peels are designed to remove the top layers of the skin, revealing fresh, new skin underneath. They can be tailored to suit different skin types and concerns, such as acne, hyperpigmentation, and fine lines. Chemical peels work by applying a blend of acids or enzymes to the skin, which causes the outer layer of skin to peel off. This process stimulates the production of collagen and elastin, leading to smoother and more youthful-looking skin.

Microdermabrasion is another effective professional skincare treatment. It involves the use of a device that uses tiny crystals or a diamond-tipped wand to exfoliate the skin gently. This process removes dead skin cells and promotes cell turnover, resulting in a smoother and more refined complexion. Microdermabrasion is particularly beneficial for reducing the appearance of acne scars, fine lines, and uneven skin texture. It also improves the absorption of skincare products, allowing them to penetrate deeper into the skin layers.

Lastly, professional skincare treatments may also include specialized treatments such as LED therapy or radiofrequency treatments. LED therapy uses different wavelengths of light to target specific skin concerns. Red light stimulates collagen production and reduces inflammation, while blue light kills acne-causing bacteria. Radiofrequency treatments, on the other hand, use radiofrequency energy to heat the deep layers of the skin. This stimulates collagen production and tightens the skin, resulting in a firmer and more youthful appearance.

Professional skincare treatments are a valuable investment in achieving and maintaining healthy and radiant skin. Whether it's a facial, chemical peel, microdermabrasion, or specialized treatments like LED therapy or radiofrequency, these treatments are performed by trained professionals who know how to address specific skin concerns effectively. By incorporating professional skincare treatments into your skincare routine, you can improve the texture, tone, and overall health of your skin for long-lasting results.

A. Overview of popular professional treatments

Popularity in professional treatments has surged in recent years, as people seek effective and convenient options to enhance their appearance and well-being. This trend can be traced back to ancient civilizations, where various beauty practices were developed and refined. These treatments, which were often reserved for the wealthy elite, have evolved over time, and gained widespread popularity in modern society.

One of the most iconic professional treatments is massage therapy. Dating back thousands of years, various forms of massage have been practiced in ancient Egypt, China, and India. These early civilizations recognized the therapeutic benefits of touch and developed techniques to alleviate pain, relax muscles, and promote overall well-being. Today, massage therapy is widely accessible in spas, wellness centers, and even hospitals, offering a range of benefits such as stress relief, improved circulation, and pain management.

Facial treatments have also played a prominent role in professional beauty practices throughout history. Ancient Egyptians were known to use natural substances like honey and milk to cleanse and moisturize their skin. In ancient Rome, wealthy individuals would indulge in luxurious facial masks made from ingredients such as egg whites and olive oil. Over time, advancements in technology and scientific research have led to the development of modern facial treatments, including chemical peels, microdermabrasion, and laser therapies. These procedures address various skin concerns, from acne to signs of aging, and have become popular for their ability to rejuvenate and transform the complexion.

For those looking to enhance their hair, professional hair treatments have become a staple in many beauty routines. Haircare practices have evolved significantly over centuries, with ancient Greeks and Romans using natural oils and herbs to nourish and style their hair. In modern times, professional hair treatments encompass a wide range of options, including keratin treatments, deep conditioning, and scalp therapies. These treatments aim to improve the health and appearance of the hair, addressing concerns such as frizz, damage, and hair loss.

Another popular professional treatment is cosmetic dentistry. Although dental health has been a concern throughout history, cosmetic dentistry has gained significant popularity in recent decades. Bright, white teeth have become synonymous with beauty and confidence. Procedures such as teeth whitening, veneers, and dental implants have become sought-after treatments, allowing individuals to enhance their smiles and improve their self-esteem.

In conclusion, the history of popular professional treatments is a fascinating journey through time. From ancient civilizations to modern society, beauty practices have evolved, and innovative treatments have emerged. Whether it's massage therapy for relaxation, facial treatments for radiant skin, hair treatments for luscious locks, or cosmetic dentistry for a dazzling smile, professional treatments have proven to be effective and popular choices for individuals seeking to enhance their appearance and well-being.

1. Facials, chemical peels, micro needling, etc.

Here's an overview of some popular professional skincare treatments:

1. **Chemical Peels:** Chemical peels involve the application of a solution to exfoliate and remove the top layer of dead skin cells. They help reduce signs of aging, improve skin texture, and treat acne and hyperpigmentation.

2. **Micro needling:** Micro needling, also known as collagen induction therapy, uses tiny needles to create controlled micro-injuries to the skin. This stimulates collagen production, improves skin texture, reduces wrinkles, and treats acne scars.

3. **Laser Therapy:** Laser treatments use focused beams of light to target specific skin issues such as wrinkles, sun damage, age spots, and acne scars. There are various types of lasers available, including ablative and non-ablative options.

4. **Microdermabrasion:** Microdermabrasion is a non-invasive treatment that uses a device to exfoliate and remove dead skin cells from the outermost layer of the skin. It helps improve skin texture, reduce fine lines, and refine pores.

5. **LED Light Therapy:** LED light therapy involves the use of different colored lights (usually red and blue) to penetrate the skin at different depths. Red light helps stimulate collagen production and reduce inflammation, while blue light targets acne-causing bacteria.

6. **HydraFacial:** HydraFacial is a multi-step facial treatment that combines exfoliation, deep cleansing, extraction, and hydration. It helps improve overall skin health, deeply cleanses pores, and provides intense hydration.

7. **Radiofrequency Skin Tightening:** This treatment uses

radiofrequency energy to heat the deeper layers of the skin, stimulating collagen production and tightening loose or sagging skin. It is commonly used to treat wrinkles, cellulite, and loose skin.

8. **Oxygen Facial:** Oxygen facials involve applying a pressurized stream of oxygen and infused serums onto the skin. This helps improve circulation, boost collagen production, and provide hydration, resulting in a brighter and healthier complexion.

It's important to note that these professional skincare treatments should be performed by trained and certified professionals. Additionally, the suitability and effectiveness of these treatments may vary depending on individual skin type and concerns.

B. When to seek professional help

Knowing when to seek professional help for your skincare needs is important for maintaining healthy skin. While there are many skincare concerns that can be addressed at home, there are situations where professional intervention is necessary.

Here are some cases when you should consider seeking professional help:

1. **Persistent skin issues:** If you have persistent acne, rosacea, eczema, psoriasis, or other chronic skin conditions, it's advisable to consult a dermatologist. They will be able to properly diagnose your condition and provide you with the most effective treatment options.

2. **Severe or sudden changes:** If you experience sudden

and severe changes in your skin like persistent redness, swelling, extreme dryness, or intense itching, it's best to see a dermatologist. These symptoms could indicate an underlying skin condition or allergic reaction that requires professional evaluation.

3. **Skin infections:** If you develop a skin infection like cellulitis, impetigo, or a fungal infection, seeking prompt medical attention is crucial. Infections may require prescription antibiotics or antifungal medication to resolve effectively.

4. **Skin cancer evaluation:** If you notice any unusual moles, growths, or spots on your skin that are changing in size, shape, color, or texture, it is important to consult a dermatologist for a thorough evaluation. Early detection and treatment of skin cancer can significantly increase the chances of successful outcomes.

5. **Skin damage or scarring:** If you have significant scarring, deep wrinkles, or facial sagging, it might be beneficial to seek professional intervention. Dermatologists and cosmetic dermatologists can offer various treatments such as laser therapy, chemical peels, or injectables to address these concerns.

6. **Skincare product reactions:** If you have a severe allergic reaction or irritation to a skincare product, discontinue its use immediately. If the symptoms persist or worsen, seek medical advice as you could be having an adverse reaction that requires medical attention.

Remember, everyone's skin is unique, and what works for one person may not work for another. Trust your instincts and seek professional help if you are unsure or concerned about your skin. Dermatologists and other skincare professionals have the expertise to provide personalized advice and treatment options for your specific needs.

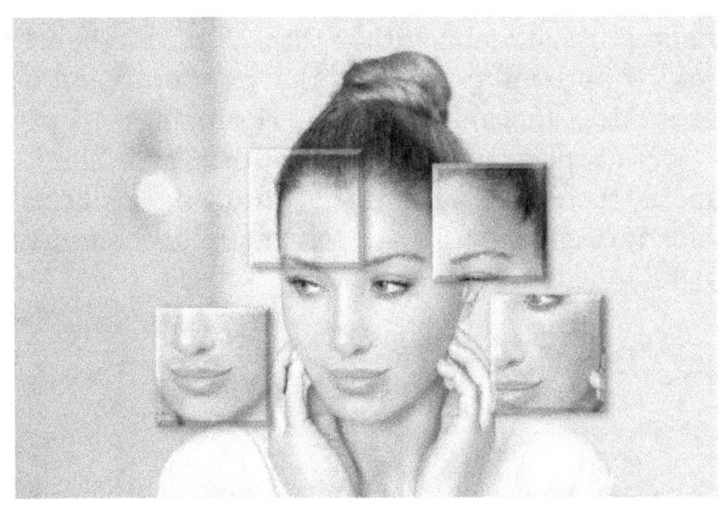

Chapter 10: Skincare for Special Situations

Skincare for special situations requires a tailored and attentive approach to address specific concerns and maintain overall skin health. One such situation is when dealing with sensitive skin. It is essential to choose gentle and fragrance-free products that won't irritate or cause inflammation. Opting for hypoallergenic cleansers, moisturizers, and sunscreens can help provide a soothing and calming effect.

For individuals with acne-prone skin, incorporating acne-fighting ingredients like salicylic acid or benzoyl peroxide can help control breakouts. Regular exfoliation can also help unclog pores and promote cell turnover. For those with dry or dehydrated skin, focusing on intense moisturization is key. Look for products that are rich in hydrating ingredients such as hyaluronic acid and ceramides.

Furthermore, individuals with aging skin can benefit from incorporating anti-aging products that contain ingredients like retinol, peptides, and antioxidants. Prioritizing sun protection by using broad-spectrum sunscreen with a high SPF is crucial in all special skincare situations. Consulting a dermatologist can provide further guidance and personalized recommendations based on individual needs.

Taking care of your skin during pregnancy is important as hormonal changes can affect your complexion.

Here are some key tips for skincare during pregnancy:

1. **Consult with your healthcare provider:** Before making any changes to your skincare routine, consult with your healthcare provider to ensure that the products you use are safe for pregnancy.

2. **Maintain a gentle skincare routine:** Stick to gentle and pregnancy-safe skincare products that are free from harsh chemicals, fragrances, and dyes. Look for skincare products labeled as "pregnancy-safe" or "safe for use during pregnancy."

3. **Stay hydrated:** Drink plenty of water to keep your skin hydrated from within. This can help prevent dryness, which is common during pregnancy.

4. **Protect from the sun:** Apply a broad-spectrum sunscreen with an SPF of 30 or higher every day to protect your skin from harmful UV rays. Wear protective clothing and seek shade when the sun is

strongest.

5. **Moisturize regularly:** Use a pregnancy-safe moisturizer to keep your skin hydrated and prevent dryness. Look for products with ingredients like hyaluronic acid, aloe vera, and shea butter, as they can help retain moisture.

6. **Avoid harsh chemicals and exfoliants:** Skip skincare products containing retinoids, salicylic acid, and hydroquinone, as they are not considered safe for use during pregnancy. Also, avoid harsh physical exfoliants that can irritate your skin.

7. **Maintain a healthy diet:** Eating a balanced diet rich in fruits, vegetables, and omega-3 fatty acids can contribute to healthy skin during pregnancy.

8. **Get enough sleep:** Prioritize getting enough sleep during pregnancy, as it can help your skin look healthier and more vibrant.

Remember, every pregnancy is different, so it's essential to consult with your healthcare provider for specific advice tailored to your needs.

B. Skincare for men

Skincare is just as important for men as it is for women.

Here are some essential skincare tips for men:

1. **Cleanse:** Start your skincare routine by using a gentle facial cleanser designed for your skin type. This will help remove dirt, oil, and impurities from your skin.

2. **Moisturize:** Moisturizer is crucial for keeping your

skin hydrated and preventing dryness. Look for a moisturizer that is lightweight and non-greasy. Apply it daily, especially after shaving.

3. **Sunscreen:** Protect your skin from the harmful effects of the sun by using a broad-spectrum sunscreen with at least SPF 30. Apply it generously on all exposed areas, including your face, neck, and hands.

4. **Exfoliate:** To remove dead skin cells and unclog pores, incorporate exfoliation into your skincare routine 2-3 times a week. Look for a facial scrub or exfoliating cleanser with gentle, non-abrasive particles.

5. **Shave with care:** Use a sharp razor and a high-quality shaving cream or gel to protect your skin from irritation, cuts, and razor burn. Shave in the direction of hair growth and rinse with cold water afterward.

6. **Eye care:** The skin around the eyes is delicate and prone to wrinkles. Invest in an eye cream or gel specifically designed to reduce puffiness, dark circles, and fine lines.

7. **Hydrate:** Drink plenty of water throughout the day to keep your skin hydrated from within. This helps maintain a healthy complexion and prevents dryness.

8. **Healthy lifestyle:** Your skincare routine is only part of the equation. Adopting a healthy lifestyle, including regular exercise, a balanced diet, and adequate sleep, can also contribute to better skin.

Remember, everyone's skin is unique, so it's important to find products that work well for you. If you have specific skincare concerns or conditions, consult a dermatologist for personalized advice.

C. Skincare for different climates

Skincare needs can vary depending on the climate you are in.

Here are some tips for taking care of your skin in different climates:

Hot and Humid Climate:

- Use a lightweight, oil-free moisturizer to avoid excessive greasiness.
- Look for products that are water-based and have a matte finish.
- Use a gentle cleanser to remove excess oil and sweat from your skin.
- Use a broad-spectrum sunscreen with a high SPF to protect your skin from harmful UV rays.
- Opt for non-comedogenic and oil-free products to prevent clogged pores and breakouts.

Cold and Dry Climate:

- Use a heavier moisturizer or hydrating cream to combat dryness and keep your skin moisturized.
- Consider using a humidifier to add moisture to the air in your living space.
- Avoid hot showers or baths, as it can strip away natural oils from your skin. Opt for lukewarm water instead.
- Apply lip balm to prevent chapped lips.
- Protect your skin with a moisturizing sunscreen, as sun damage can still occur in cold climates.

- Hydrate your skin by using a moisturizer that provides both hydration and sun protection.

- Wear lightweight, breathable clothing that covers your skin, or use a broad-brimmed hat, sunglasses, and an umbrella to protect yourself from the sun's rays.

- Apply a broad-spectrum sunscreen with a high SPF regularly, especially on exposed areas.

- Keep your skin hydrated by drinking plenty of water and using a hydrating facial mist throughout the day.

Windy Climate:

- Protect your skin by using a heavier moisturizer or balm to create a barrier against the wind.

- Wear protective clothing, such as scarves or hats, to shield your skin from the wind.

- Apply lip balm with SPF to protect your lips.

- Use a gentle cleanser and avoid harsh exfoliants or scrubs that can further irritate your skin.

- Moisturize your skin frequently, especially after being exposed to the wind.

Remember, everyone's skin is unique, so it's essential to listen to your skin and adjust your skincare routine accordingly. If you experience any severe skin issues or concerns, it's advisable to consult a dermatologist for personalized advice.

Conclusion

In this book, we have explored the fascinating world of skincare and uncovered the secrets to achieving healthier, more radiant skin.

Let's take a moment to recap the key points we have discussed:

We discussed the importance of understanding your skin type and its specific needs. Every individual has a unique skin type, whether it is oily, dry, combination, or sensitive. By identifying your skin type, you can tailor your skincare routine and choose products that address your specific concerns.

We then delved into the essential steps of a skincare routine, which include cleansing, exfoliating, toning, moisturizing, and protecting. These steps, when performed consistently and with the right products, can greatly boost the health and appearance of your skin.

We also explored the importance of nourishing our skin from within through a balanced diet, hydration, and lifestyle choices. Our skin reflects our overall health, and by taking care of our bodies, we indirectly take care of our skin as well.

Furthermore, we discussed the impact of external factors such as pollution, sun exposure, and stress on our skin. We emphasized the importance of protecting our skin with sunscreen, antioxidants, and stress management techniques.

Now that we have covered these key points, it is crucial to reinforce the importance of consistency. Skincare is not a one-time task; it is an ongoing commitment. Results are realized over time, and by sticking to a regular skincare routine, you can achieve long-lasting improvements in the health and appearance of your skin.

So, my final words of encouragement to you are to be patient and keep going. There may be moments when you want to give up or when you don't see immediate results but remember that great skin takes time and dedication. Each day that you stick to your skincare routine, you are investing in the future of your skin.

Your skin reflects your self-care and self-love, and by maintaining consistent skincare habits, you are sending a message to yourself and others that you value your well-being. Remember to embrace the process, enjoy the journey, and indulge in the self-care rituals that make you feel beautiful and confident.

So go ahead, start each day with love and care for your skin, and watch as it blossoms into its healthiest and most radiant state. Your skin deserves the best, and you have the power to give it just that through a consistent skincare routine.

Resources

BOOKS:

1. **"The Skin Type Solution"** by Leslie Baumann

2. **"The Little Book of Skin Care: Korean Beauty Secrets for Healthy, Glowing Skin"** by Charlotte Cho

3. **"Skin Rules: Trade Secrets from a Top New York Dermatologist"** by Debra Jaliman

4. **"The Beauty of Dirty Skin: The Surprising Science of Looking and Feeling Radiant from the Inside Out"** by Whitney Bowe

5. **"Simple Skin Beauty: Every Woman's Guide to a Lifetime of Healthy, Gorgeous Skin"** by Ellen Marmur

ONLINE RESOURCES:

1. **American Academy of Dermatology (AAD):** Their website offers a wealth of information on skincare, covering various topics like acne, aging skin, sun protection, and more. Visit: https://www.aad.org/public

2. **WebMD Skin Health Center:** Provides comprehensive information on various skin conditions, treatments, and general skincare tips. Visit: https://www.webmd.com/skin-problems-and-treatments/default.htm

3. **Paula's Choice Skincare:** This website offers extensive information on skincare ingredients, product

reviews, and research-backed advice. Visit: https://www.paulaschoice.com/expert-advice

4. **DermNet NZ:** A dermatology resource with an extensive collection of information on various skin conditions, including photos, treatment options, and patient education materials. Visit: https://dermnetnz.org/

5. **SkincareAddiction (Reddit):** A community-driven platform where members share tips, product recommendations, and skincare routines. Visit: https://www.reddit.com/r/SkincareAddiction/

ASSOCIATIONS:

1. **American Academy of Dermatology (AAD):** A professional association of dermatologists that provides resources, education, and research in the field of dermatology. Visit: https://www.aad.org/

2. **European Academy of Dermatology and Venereology (EADV):** A non-profit organization aiming to advance research and education in dermatology and venereology. Visit: https://www.eadvsymposium2021.org/

3. **International Society of Dermatology (ISD):** A global organization promoting excellence in dermatology education, research, and patient care. Visit: https://www.intsocderm.org/

Please note that while these resources can provide valuable information, it is always important to consult a licensed dermatologist or healthcare professional for personalized advice and diagnosis.

Research

Research Articles:

Kim, M. E., Cho, S., Lee, Y. M., & Kim, D. (2020). Role of skin care in the prevention of skin aging. Annals of dermatology, 32(1), 1-10.

Rawlings, A. V. (2004). Trends in stratum corneum research and the management of dry skin conditions. International Journal of Cosmetic Science, 26(2), 63-95.

Farage, M. A., Katsarou, A., & Maibach, H. I. (2008). Sensory, clinical, and physiological factors in sensitive skin: a review. Contact Dermatitis, 58(2), 129-140.

Draelos, Z. D. (2010). Cosmeceuticals for aging skin. Clinics in Dermatology, 28(6), 597-603.

Godic, A., Poljšak, B., Adamic, M., & Dahmane, R. (2014). The role of antioxidants in skin cancer prevention and treatment. Oxidative Medicine and Cellular Longevity, 2014.

Books:

Baumann, L. (2009). Cosmeceuticals and Cosmetic Ingredients (1st ed.). McGraw-Hill Education.

Draelos, Z. D. (2014). Cosmeceuticals (3rd ed.). Elsevier.

Bouloc, A., & Rakotobe, S. (2016). The Skin and Cosmetics Ingredients Dictionary (2nd ed.). Allured Books.

Loden, M., & Maibach, H. I. (2000). Dry Skin and Moisturizers: Chemistry and Function (2nd ed.). CRC Press.

Del Rosso, J. Q. (2013). The Hydration Prescription: Healing Your Skin from the Inside Out. Healthy Skin Press.

Bibliography

Baumann, L., & Saghari, S. (2017). Skin ageing and its treatment. Journal of Pathology, 241(4), 457-464.

Farage, M. A., Miller, K. W., Elsner, P., & Maibach, H. I. (2008). Characteristics of the aging skin. Advances in Wound Care, 21(6), 247-261.

Rawlings, A. V. (2006). Trends in stratum corneum research and the management of dry skin conditions. International Journal of Cosmetic Science, 28(3), 157-167.

Fisher, G. J., Kang, S., Varani, J., Bata-Csorgo, Z., & Wan, Y. (2002). Mechanisms of photoaging and chronological skin aging. Archives of Dermatology, 138(11), 1462-1470.

Wickett, R. R., Visscher, M. O., & Wu, Y. (2009). Transepidermal water loss and skin surface pH in infant skin treated with cleansers and infant wipes. Journal of Clinical Pediatrics, 48(Supplement 3), 15S-21S.

Kligman, A. M., & Grove, G. L. (1985). Regulation of sebaceous gland activity by sex steroids. Dermato-Endocrinology, 22(1), 19-25.

Rittié, L., & Fisher, G. J. (2015). Natural and sun-induced aging of human skin. Cold Spring Harbor Perspectives in Medicine, 5(1), a015370.

Farage, M. A., & Miller, K. W. (2013). Elsner, physiology of the skin, third edition: Georg von Mackensen, MD et al. P & S, 22(2), 133-134.

Pillai, S., Oresajo, C., & Hayward, J. (2005). Ultraviolet radiation and skin aging: roles of reactive oxygen species, inflammation and protease activation, and strategies for prevention of inflammation-induced matrix degradation - a review. International Journal of Cosmetic Science, 27(1), 17-34.

Farage, M. A., Katsarou, A., & Maibach, H. I. (2007). Sensory, clinical, and physiological factors in sensitive skin: a review. Contact Dermatitis, 57(2), 87-94.

"The Little Book of Skin Care: Korean Beauty Secrets for Healthy, Glowing Skin" by Charlotte Cho

"The Skincare Bible: Your No-Nonsense Guide to Great Skin" by Dr. Anjali Mahto

"The Beauty of Dirty Skin: The Surprising Science of Looking and Feeling Radiant from the Inside Out" by Whitney Bowe, MD

"The Skin Nerd: Your Straight-Talking Guide to Feeding, Protecting and Respecting Your Skin" by Jennifer Rock

"Skin Rules: Trade Secrets from a Top New York Dermatologist" by Debra Jaliman, MD

"The Little Book of Big Beauty: Beyond Flawless Skin and Bouncy Hair, Real Sketches of Real Beauty" by LaTonya Goffney

"The Japanese Skincare Revolution: How to Have the Most Beautiful Skin of Your Life - at Any Age" by Chizu Saeki and Hirokazu Takayama

"Clean Skin from Within: The Spa Doctor's Two-Week Program to Glowing, Naturally Youthful Skin" by Trevor Cates, ND

"Skin: A Biography" by Sharad P. Paul, MD

"Pretty Honest: The Straight-Talking Beauty Companion" by Sali Hughes

"Skin Deep: Women on Skin Care, Makeup, and Looking Their

Best" edited by Bee Shapiro

"**Younger: The Breakthrough Anti-Aging Method for Radiant Skin**" by Harold Lancer, MD

"**The Healthy Skin Diet: Your Complete Guide to Beautiful Skin in Only 8 Weeks!**" by Karen Fischer

"**The Beauty Geek's Guide to Skin Care: 1,000 Essential Definitions of Common Product Ingredients**" by Deborah Burnes

"**The Skin Type Solution: A Revolutionary Guide to Your Best Skin Ever**" by Leslie Baumann, MD

"**In My Skin: A Memoir of Addiction**" by Kate Holden

"**The Essential Guide to Aging Skin: How to Keep Your Skin Beautiful and Radiant in Your 40s, 50s, 60s and Beyond**" by Dr. Ellie Nadelson

"**The Little Book of Skin Care for Men: A Simple Guide to Looking Good at Any Age**" by Rocky Angelucci

"**The Beauty Myth: How Images of Beauty Are Used Against Women**" by Naomi Wolf

"**Ageless Beauty: The Secrets to French Elegance and Timeless Chic**" by Clémence von Mueffling

About The Author

Kimberly Hodge

Kimberly is a retired health and wellness career college instructor whose focus of writing is on health, wellness, and business topics. When not writing she spends her time with her husband and fur baby on the east coast of the United States.

Books By This Author

Cosmetics: Secrets & Tips

In the world of beauty, secrets lie within the transformative power of cosmetics. From the pursuit of flawless skin to enhancing one's natural features, "Cosmetics: Secrets and Tips," is a guide that delves into the realms of makeup artistry. This book is a treasury of insider knowledge, curated for anyone who yearns to discover the secrets behind the enchanting allure of cosmetics.

Inside these pages, readers will embark on a journey through the rich history of beauty, exploring the evolution of makeup from ancient civilizations to contemporary trends. Unravel the mysteries behind selecting the right foundation, the nuances of highlighting and contouring, and the secrets to achieving the perfect cat-eye or smoky eye effect.

With insightful advice, easy-to-follow techniques, and a celebration of diversity, this book will empower readers to express themselves authentically while unveiling their true beauty potential. Prepare to embark on an extraordinary beauty journey with "Cosmetics Secrets and Tips" and discover the secrets that will unveil your inner radiance.

Bath And Body Business: A Girl's Guide To Starting A Homebased Business

Bath and Body Business: A Girl's Guide to Starting a Homebased Business

This book was written by an experienced business owner who shares her creative path to starting a successful business from home. You will learn the basics to get you up and running quickly and efficiently.

Topics Discussed:

Business Plans
Licensing
Insurance
Labeling Requirements
Business Management
Product Pricing
Social Media Marketing
Bookkeeping
Goal Setting
Time Management
Recipes
Wholesale Suppliers
and Much More!

In addition, you will find resources to online courses, professional small business tax information, and small business development.

Manifesting Happiness: A Practical Guide To Transforming Your Life

After reading this practical guide, you will find that you, too, can lead a life of happiness! Embrace the power within you to transform your existence into an exhilarating journey filled with joy and fulfillment. Unlock the secret sauce of happiness and let it permeate every aspect of your being, igniting a fire in your heart that burns brighter than ever before.

With each turn of the page, you'll discover invaluable tools and techniques that empower you to create a life that resonates with excitement and positivity. From fostering meaningful relationships to nurturing self-love, from pursuing passions relentlessly to finding gratitude in even the smallest moments - this guide unravels all the mysteries behind cultivating genuine happiness.

No longer will it be elusive or unattainable; instead, it will become a vibrant reality pulsating through your veins. The world is brimming with endless possibilities waiting for you to seize them; grab hold of life's adventure and savor every delicious moment on this thrilling path toward everlasting bliss!

Simply Handmade: Beauty & Skincare Handcrafted Recipes

Interest in handmade all-natural beauty and skincare products has grown enormously in the last few years. More and more health-conscious people are realizing the harmful effects of chemical-laden beauty and bath products on the skin.

Thankfully, there are solutions for safer, more affordable, and most importantly, all-natural handmade products for you to make at home!

In this book, you'll discover the incredible health benefits of creating your own all-natural beauty and skincare products, as well as, many recipes to whip up luscious products of your own to enjoy!

Easy-To-Make Products, Including:

Bath Bombs
Body Butters

Bath Salts
Sugar Scrubs
Hair Care Products
Lip Balms & Scrubs
Healing Salves
Homemade Laundry Detergent
Solid Perfumes
Room Refresher Sprays
And many more!

Imperfect: A Path To Self Loving

Welcome to a journey of self-discovery, acceptance, and love. In a world that constantly bombards us with images of perfection and unattainable standards, it's easy to feel lost or inadequate.

But what if we told you that embracing your imperfections could lead you on the path to self-love? It's time to break free from society's expectations and embark on a beautiful journey toward accepting and celebrating your unique self.

In this book, we'll delve into why loving your imperfect self is crucial and liberating. We'll explore practical ways to treat yourself with kindness and compassion as you navigate through life's ups and downs. And most importantly, we'll guide you in discovering how your perfect imperfections can be the catalyst for authenticity.

So grab a cup of tea (or coffee if that's more your style), get comfortable, and let's dive into the wonderful world of embracing imperfection as our pathway toward true self-love.